# AT THE PRECIPICE

# AT THE PRECIPICE

## My Three-Year Journey from Stroke to Good Health with Type 2 Diabetes

Jim Snell

iUniverse, Inc.
Bloomington

# AT THE PRECIPICE
## My Three-Year Journey from Stroke to Good Health with Type 2 Diabetes

iUniverse books may be ordered through booksellers or by contacting:

iUniverse
1663 Liberty Drive
Bloomington, IN 47403
www.iuniverse.com
1-800-Authors (1-800-288-4677)

ISBN: 978-1-4620-3456-7 (sc)
ISBN: 978-1-4620-3458-1 (ebk)

Library of Congress Control Number: 2011910497

Printed in the United States of America

iUniverse rev. date: 08/08/2011

# CONTENTS

# Preface

I wrote this book to share my experiences and detail how, after thirty years of my blood glucose numbers being all over the map, followed by a stroke on December 2, 2007, and serious degradation of my body by diabetes I was able to correct the situation to manage my type 2 diabetes properly for the first time. This stroke affected my balance, knocked my right eye out of alignment, gave me partial right-side paralysis, and hindered my ability to walk properly. This is not a self-help book, nor do I recommend that you follow the techniques, schedules, or medicines I used. Your medical regimen plan needs to be thoroughly reviewed, discussed, and approved by your doctor before you make any changes.

Occurrences of diabetes have exploded in America and elsewhere. This means a huge amount of time, cost, and effort are needed to combat the disease. Doctors must see more and more patients in shorter and shorter time intervals. The goal of this book is twofold: first, to reduce the chances that others will have a stroke like or worse than the one I had; second, to share information about diabetes and show readers how to help their doctors and diabetic trainers manage their care. The best way to do this is to learn about the disease and collect the data that will get the targeted care that is needed.

When someone goes to a doctor, often the generic advice is to focus on three main issues and solve them in that short visit. In fact, a diabetic patient, especially a new one, may have a tractor-trailer load of valid questions that all take priority, and he or she may feel overwhelmed.

My hope is that this book will give you insight, hope, and ideas that you can review with your doctor to improve your type

2 diabetes program. I have tried to provide detailed explanations (written for the layman) of how things work, what I bumped into when working with my doctor, how we solved problems that arose, and the day-to-day management of my type 2 diabetes. My goal is to reduce the steep learning curve on this disease and its management from a layman's perspective, to shine a light on it, and to ensure others don't have to spend the three-plus years of grief I went through to get this under control.

In the early stages of type 2 diabetes detection, it may seem you can take shortcuts, reduce intake of carbohydrates, cut out all extra candy and sugars, and proceed. I am here to tell you—don't kid yourself, and follow your doctor's medical, diet, measurement, and exercise advice closely. Should you have questions and confusion, it is most important to resolve those early and quickly. That is where one can quickly get off track and lost.

Lastly, I need to send my deepest heartfelt thanks to my wife, Sharon, and my medical team (all located in California) for their unstinting help and care, in particular:

Dr. Wilson Fung, MD, head doctor and diabetes doctor, Camarillo

Dr. Phillip E. Maurice, MD, neurologist, Thousand Oaks

Dr. Susan Chang, MD, kidney doctor, Camarillo

Dr. Lewis Kanter, MD, allergy and lungs, Coastal Allergy Care, Camarillo

James B. Mayer, OD, FCOVD, specialists in strabismus and repair of double vision, Agape Optometry and Learning Center, Thousand Oaks

Dr. Kenneth R. Diddie, MD, retina specialist, Westlake Village

Grace Wong, Pharmacist/Owner - Medicine Shoppe Newberry Park. Ca.

St. Johns Hospital and Rehab Ward, Oxnard

Best wishes and good luck.

James W. Snell
April 2011

# Chapter 1

## Introduction

The last few weeks have seen clear evidence of my last three-plus years, struggling to effect an incredible turnaround of my type 2 diabetes and get it under better control.

On Sunday, November 7, 2010, I ran a Bayer At Home A1CNOW test to evaluate my A1C number, which was an amazing 6.9 percent. According to the documentation in the kit, 6.9 is in the green zone called "in control." It was a remarkable improvement. A prior test done a year or so earlier had been horrific, with a reading of 13.3 percent. The A1C number is a measurement of the blood sugar glucose that has been picked up by the blood hemoglobin and provides a three-month history of the levels that one's blood has been at.

In October 2010, a lab test of my kidneys showed all good numbers in range and spec, and their efficiency had changed direction and now were showing improvement. My eye doctor noticed that my retinas were no longer hemorrhaging and had shown extensive healing. My allergist confirmed that my lungs had been improving. He put me on his gas analyzer laboratory machine. In the past, I could barely blow 470 with the aid of Albuterol and Qvar inhalers. Now I could easily blow 520 or better without aid on the handheld volume check unit.

Finally, thanks to a twelve hundred-calorie diet, I have seen my weight drop dramatically—from a high of 330 pounds down to

280, and it is still dropping. Previously, I could not lose a pound, no matter what I did.

In January 2011, I obtained a Continuous Glucose Monitor System (CGMS) so I could conduct my readings without sticking my finger thirty-two times a day. One month later, I was walking faster and better and started having serious hypoglycemic moments that required me to reduce my medication that included needle insulin type and pills. The comments out there indicate one can gain tighter control of diabetes by using a CGMS. That has been my experience.

After a three-year-plus journey, starting with my stroke on December 2, 2007, and through four distinct phases of healing, I am now on the correct path, and my type 2 diabetes is under control. I had been detected as a type 2 diabetic in the 1980s and have been fighting that all the way through to today.

The first phase took a year; this was the recuperating from the stroke, dealing with the physical disabilities it caused, and fixing my broken binocular vision. My right side, including my right eye, and balance on that side, was affected.

The second phase lasted another year. I struggled with my diabetes, with horrendous blood glucose (BG) numbers and daily high numbers every morning, and excess water in my lower extremities and constant water weeping from both legs without a known cause. Extensive BG numbers were taken and logged by me, and I walked two miles per day every day and made my first attempts to eat a twelve hundred-calorie diet. I had a scrotum filled with fluid; it was like a large cannonball. I took diuretics to get the excess water out.

The third phase began when my doctors concluded that the "liver dawn effect" and "emergency glucose addition effect" were broken due to failed hormonal communications between the gut, pancreas, and liver, which resulted in massive glucose increases from the liver (278–380 units). *Note:* The liver dawn effect is the role played by your liver to add sugar to your body just before you wake up, so that you are prepared to start the day. As long as the signaling between your pancreas (which generates the insulin) and liver (which regulates the insulin present in the blood) is working, the liver will add the correct amount of glucose. If not, your system will get a full-pail load of glucose, as though it is preparing you for the French Foreign Legion starvation march across the Sahara.

An emergency liver glucose addition is commonly called a "liver dump." When the pancreas-liver signaling is working properly, this glucose addition by the liver is invisible and should not inflate your blood glucose through the roof (i.e., from 278–311 or higher).

If one does not eat or at those times when the gut has no glucose to add, the liver dump occurs. The liver's role is to provide glucose and keep one's brain and cells alive. When the gut is providing glucose, the liver is supposed to be in fasting phase. When the gut has no more glucose to provide, the liver is supposed to switch to its sugar-making mode and supply glucose from its emergency supply. Researchers suggest that in type 2 diabetes the liver is always in sugar-making mode and does not return to the fasting mode when it is supposed to.

Around May 2010, after I researched this issue online, my doctors agreed that I should take additional metformin pills—500 milligrams (mg) at 10:00 p.m. and 12:00 a.m.—to shut down the dawn effect from midnight till 5:30 a.m. In addition, I was to aggressively monitor my BG and prevent it from going below 100 and triggering an emergency liver dump–glucose add. I adjusted my low-glycemic diet to ensure I had sufficient carbohydrates, which would generate the necessary glucose to keep my body and its cells running. (The alternatives are to take glucose tablets or accept that one's liver will be forced to keep releasing extra glucose and hope it is a controlled release and not one that blasts your BG averages off the map.)

The last phase was the use of a Continuous Glucose Monitor System (CGMS), which was not expected to be difficult but was a key change due to the information I'd gained by actively monitoring my BG twenty-four hours a day, seven days a week. In this phase, there was a dramatic change in needle insulin type, a large reduction in the doses, and the removal of the insulin-activating drug Starlix. I saw quite a stable running of the body's BG, similar to what most folks have, where it is slowly changing like waves on a placid lake. My numbers had been all over the place for the previous thirty years.

Finally, I continued my multi-loop, quarter-mile walking program every day and added extra walks when the BG was 190 or higher.

The result is documented above: the November 7, 2010, A1C of 6.9. The stroke had caused the loss of my job; mechanical, perseverance, and optical deficiencies; and disabilities that prevented the tools of my profession. It took me three-plus years to clean up this mess and get back on track. As best as I can tell tell from all the discussion out there, this disease has common factors at the highest level, having to do with carbohydrate control, diet, and hearty exercise. The aging and degradation of the endocrine system affects everyone slightly differently and in many ways that makes everyone's case different and difficult to treat.

For clarity, it needs pointing out that type 1 diabetes is generally considered to be an insulin failure by the pancreas and immediate treatment is needle insulin. Type 2 is a catch-all including everyone who is not type 1 but has excess, poorly controlled glucose in their body for a host of reasons. This is not a full list, but many reasons include reduced insulin generation by the pancreas; reduced meal bolus by pancreas; reduced basal insulin by pancreas; excess glucose production by liver; too many carbohydrates in meals; insufficient exercise; insulin resistance; etc.

The other great difficulty in dealing with a debilitating, sneaky disease like type 2 diabetes is that it has so many symptoms, and pinpointing the fix is complex and time-consuming. Our medical system is better geared to solving "battlefield injuries" (e.g., to size up a patient in as little time as possible, get the—eureka!—best first guess, and send the patient home with pills and the doctor's orders).

It takes hours and extensive data for any experts assisting in your care to really help you. A three- to five-minute conversation in the office of a doctor pressured to see as many patients as possible in the shortest time interval will have poor success without your detailed help and involvement. You will need to learn about and investigate the disease and current thinking about its cure, preferably online. Online gives one faster and broader access to the latest medical reports, and many good websites specialize in diabetes care and diagnosis. You have to be prepared to monitor your disease and take blood glucose readings, control your carbohydrates, and maintain your diet and exercise routines. Only you can do that. When you do this, you will get the detailed knowledge and data your team of experts—doctor, dietitian, endocrinologist, and diabetes trainer, etc.—need to quickly and efficiently help you tie this monster down. This is also the key to maintaining good long-term health, vision, body, kidneys, limbs, and a healthy heart. Of course, your doctor will identify the medications you need for insulin generation as you age. All can be resolved with a viable plan and approach.

Another serious concern is that type 2 diabetes is constantly changing its spots; it can be affected by weather, disease, colds, emotions, and aging. One has to watch and be prepared for flexibility and adaption. Even I was shocked when, after I completed the first draft of this book in November 2010, I went out and got a continuous glucose monitor and found that my body—through exercise and diet control—had changed. I needed to cut back on the oral insulin-generating drugs: instead of Starlix and the type of needle insulin called Humalog 75/25 at 23 units once a day in the morning, I started taking Humalog standard Lispro: four units in the morning, three at lunch, and three at dinner. I'd thought I would simply add better and more detailed data monitoring and roll along. Nope, after three years of working on this, the medicine changed for the better, but it took a lot of effort and patience to modify the program. My diet stayed the same and the hearty daily exercise continued unabated. If you get detected early enough, simple changes in diet and exercise can obviate the need for more aggressive management. If you are a strong, type A personality like I am, if your brain can ramp your heart rate up (160 to 190 on BP and rate of 120 or higher) when you are seriously thinking about an issue, or your natural fight-or flight-body response is set off and puts you on a DEFCON 5 level at the slightest of provocation—look out. Your blood glucose can change easily and quickly all over the map and will need very frequent and proactive monitoring.

You'll need to ask yourself three questions (discussed in detail later): Do you have a relatively stable BG level that slowly moves up and down in response to the food you've eaten?

Are your dawn effect and emergency liver glucose addition effects working reasonably well and not adding too much glucose? If not, your A1C number will be a clue. It will be above eight; mine was 13.3. Another clue will come from your blood-glucose meter readings, which could be as high as 150 at 3:00 a.m. and 200-plus by breakfast.Do you know your body's pill-ingestion times, the up-to-strength live time of the pill, and the body exit time? This is to ensure you have proper glucose as well as blood pressure all day long, until bedtime, when taking your recommended medicines, including heart pills, etc.

If the answers are stable glucose waveforms; no problem with the liver and its glucose functions and buffering; and your A1C is under control, you will find a lot of what follows to be interesting reading. You can drop blood testing to four to six strips a day, whatever your doctor recommends. (Anything you do to care for your diabetes must be reviewed and approved by your diabetes doctor, without exception.) Otherwise, you will want to read all chapters in this book thoroughly.

Finally, I leave you with this paraphrase from a TV commercial:

So you have been diagnosed with type 2 diabetes. You may choose to feel sorry for yourself. I hope you don't. I hope you find a good doctor and learn something about your body and diabetes. You'll need to go on a simple diet coupled with a good exercise program. Last, you'll need to learn how to use a blood-glucose meter, and test often.

# Chapter 2

## Phase 1: The Stroke

The first sign that something was deadly off track occurred in the wee hours of Sunday, December 2, 2007, as I crawled upstairs to the master bedroom. The next thing I remember was pain and a buzzing in my head, and I found myself on the floor. I crawled back to bed. I could not sit up or balance on my right. My face muscles were all sagging on the right side. I told my wife to call an ambulance. When I arrived at the St. John's Hospital emergency room, a doctor pestered me, asking when exactly this (i.e., the stroke) had happened. He needed to know so he could administer a special drug to clear the stroke. I honestly could not tell him. It turned out that my blood pressure was 210. I do not have the low number, as the higher number was the critical one in this case, and I might have bled to death on the operating table if I'd taken that drug.

The drug was not administered. Instead, I was given aspirin and kept in the emergency ward for two days for observation. Then I was moved to a regular hospital ward, where the doctors attempted to see if I could stand or walk. Fortunately, all seemed to be working—arms, hands, legs, toes, voice, eyes, brain, etc. The doctors did a CAT scan and MRI of my brain, upper chest, and heart. The CAT scan was clean; the MRI found a small clot issue in the area of my brain to do with right-side balance, movement, and eyesight. Nothing else seemed to be affected. In addition, an ultrasound of my heart and blood vessels found no evidence of any floating debris or minor clots. They checked my voice box, and no problems or paralysis were found.

However, my right-side balance was blown. A damaged nerve feeding my right eye meant that my binocular vision was not working; instead, I saw two independent images. There also was some paralysis on the right side. I could not detect differences in temperature with my left hand; when I picked up ice with my left hand, I couldn't feel the cold, which was dangerous. The right hand was good; touch and feel were functional. And I couldn't stand or walk.

I was sent over to a rehab group at the main branch of St. John's Hospital to relearn walking and standing as well as exercise the muscles that had been hit by the stroke. After thirty days in the hospital, I finally could walk with a walker and make it once around the nursing offices and rehab ward. I spent most of my time exercising and wheeling myself around in a wheelchair. I was not permitted to move on two feet without assistance and supervision.

Before I could be released and sent home, my bathroom had to be modified with support rods, a toilet chair, and a shower bench so I could move myself around. My son came from Bothell, Washington, and set up my bathroom. Because I could not walk up and down the stairs to the master bedroom, I had to have a bed set up downstairs in my small den. This bed did not have side safety rails like a hospital bed, so I would roll out onto the floor when asleep and hurt myself. (Now I sleep in a recliner that keeps me locked in.)

I spent most of my time using my walker and sleeping, trying to recover from stroke. Two or three hours of effort, and I was dead. Going back to work as a working/managing director of an electronics hardware engineering team designing ADSL2 and fiber to the home and new-age telephony gear based on Internet technology was out of the question.

My double vision drove me nuts, and regular optometrists were no help. After searching around I found a special group of optometrists who deal with strabismus eye problems and related deficiencies. As it turned out, they were a godsend and were able to isolate an eye-nerve paralysis that was affecting my vision, even though both eyes could move and track. They discovered that a prism of the correct strength could return some of my binocular vision. Reading books, newspaper columns, and fine-print documents is still very difficult and requires a large electronic magnifier and lamp of six diopter magnification. I used to love to read, and now it is an effort at all times.

It usually takes a year to recover from a stroke, and sometimes recovery does not happen as the body attempts to plumb around the blockage. My vision and right-side balance never recovered, and I still wear special glasses to correct my right-eye vision. My thinking brain now takes care of both balance and walking; there's no double-tasking like in past. After two years, my reptilian-central cortex brain is now helping me to learn to drive again. I say "reptilian" because of the response time: the reptilian/central cortex brain responds in 30 milliseconds, the thinking brain, 140 milliseconds. Fighter pilot simulator training involves training the central cortex to make the fastest critical decisions automatically without thinking about it and the delays involved.

I tried to control my diabetes but was not very successful during this time. The best I did was to better record BG numbers, which were terrible in the morning, and I was unclear how to proceed. The best I could do was to fix my vision, work on legal/disability issues, struggle to walk longer and better, and improve my strength.

# Chapter 3

# Phase 2: Working through the Diabetes and Other Problems

After struggling through my recovery for a year and gaining strength, I felt it was time to focus on my diabetes. During this time, my kidney doctor wanted to remove Actos from my list of medications, the only drug that was getting the BG numbers down to a minimum of 185 and no lower starting from 240 plus.

My body was degenerating due the severe diabetes and resulting in excessive weight. My legs were swollen with extra water and weeping, and my scrotum had filled up with water and looked like a huge cannonball. The only way to get my BG down under 185 was to exercise very strongly, and this was two miles. I started walking around my condo park in quarter-mile loops and noticed that five loops in the morning did not drop my BG. Usually, only after six or eight loops (two miles) would my BG drop to 100 by 10:00 a.m. Each and every morning was the same.

My doctor and kidney doctor were working on my water issues; my kidney numbers were not great, and renal efficiency was decreasing. The kidney doctor added more diuretics and that showed promise in getting the fluid out. In all, eighteen pounds of water were removed. Finally, my scrotum shrank back to normal. (I had made a number of visits to a surgeon and other doctors, who checked me out for hernia, but a CAT scan confirmed there was water in my scrotum.) The big question was: where in the devil was all the fluid coming from? The answer was there was way too much glucose in my blood system because of an errant liver, and my body was attempting to dilute it. There was still something serious going on, but the exercise got my BG down to one hundred. With a simple diet and portion control, it was possible to keep it under control until midnight, but the next morning my liver would hammer my body again.

I set up a 1,200-calorie diet and restricted alcohol. It was to no avail; my morning BG numbers still pounded out at 238-plus, with no exception. It took almost a year for me to tame this right down, when I learned about the liver-dump functions of dawn effect and other dumps that occur when the body is running short of glucose.

# Chapter 4

# Phase 3: Solving the Issues

More than a year ago, I discovered that the way to get the morning 238 BG back to 100 or thereabouts on the BG meter in morning was to walk minimum of two miles, or eight times around the condo park. A number of times from midnight to 6:00 a.m., I had logged blood-sugar readings such as: 1:00 a.m.–110; 3:00 a.m.–150; 6:00 a.m.–234 to 280. Prior to midnight, my BG would be around 100. This is how you trap an errant liver; the endocrine system loads you up with excessive glucose. The liver works on a inverse feedback system that looks at the insulin in the blood and assumes if it cannot see any insulin due to either no insulin or faulty sensing, the liver assumes one needs more sugar and proceeds to add glucose to blood until it sees the insulin. In my case that meant a huge dump of glucose.

I stopped eating, went on a restrictive diet; still, the numbers would not go down until I'd walked two miles. This occurred each morning, every day, without fail. I asked numerous medical people why but got no rational answer. One told me that my metabolism was slow to start.

Food had no effect on this nonsense; at least, it never brought it down. One item was clear; once the two-mile walk was done, my sugar level dropped and finally got back to 100. Otherwise, my levels stayed stuck at 180-plus, no exception. It was most frustrating. I even saw an endocrinologist, at the request of my kidney doctor.

That proved to be insulting; the endocrinologist was berating and useless. Notwithstanding that I was trying to clean up the mess and get back on track with the best of help, and I found my way to the new doctor's office.

I kept looking up issues on websites and finally found some interesting data about the dawn and "Somogyi" effects—services of the liver in which glucose gets stuffed into the blood system. In a normal body, these functions should result only in glucose adds that do not overwhelm system.

As stated earlier, the dawn effect is the wakeup morning services by liver to add glucose for startup of the body. There are other liver dumps that are not a result of too little glucose and result from some disturbances in the body BG when levels are dropping due to gut emptying and then the BG quickly starts back up due to some more food following quickly behind the main meal. I have observed these phenomena many times on the CGMS and repeated with testing and caught sympathetic liver dumps by liver when BG was fine and in levels from 140 to 200. For reasons that escape me, I have seen dumps that occur when the fingertip BG is 150 to 200, the gut is emptying, and the BG is slowly dropping; when a snack is added, the liver will hop in and do a dump. I have watched and logged these events. I have read comments online that indicate that in some folks these functions are totally disruptive and some say are psychosomatic and caused by the brain.

Fortunately, a few isolated comments also revealed that some folks were using shots of basal insulin and metformin pills at night. Basal insulin is the insulin that the body releases constantly to keep body and functions running and there are commercial equivalents of basal insulin. One night I fell asleep and forgot to take my dinnertime metformin. I took it at midnight and was surprised to get reduced morning BG reading. I checked with my primary-care doctor, and he prescribed a 500 mg tablet at 10:00 p.m. and one at midnight. This blocked off the dawn effect from midnight to 5:00 a.m. My BG at midnight was 108, and at 5:00 a.m. it was 103.

A word to the wise: the liver appears to block the glucose add action while metformin is up to strength in the blood system. In my case, the pills take two and a half hours to get into the system, last two hours, and leave in half an hour. After 5:30 a.m., when the midnight pill wears off, the liver pumps the blood system, trying to bring glucose up. How did I resolve this? I take a breakfast metformin pill at 5:00 a.m., shoot up 23 units of Humalog, wait one hour for the Humalog to get into my system, and then take one to three quarter-mile walks. The 5:00 a.m. metformin starts making its presence known by 7:30 a.m.; the Humalog and the walks beat down the extra glucose; and the liver, corralled back into its cage, stops sending out sugar. If my morning sugar is 120 or less, one quarter-mile walk is sufficient. If my BG is 170, then three walks are sufficient.

In February 2011, when the insulin type/dose was revised and metformin timing altered slightly, the process was modified to take 4 units of Humalog Lispro Insulin at 5:30 am; metformin pill and other pills at 6:15 am; breakfast at 6:30 am and walks started at 7:30 am. Results were excellent as well on change.

Some of you may be asking: what does all this "standing on one's head, drinking a glass of water" prove? The answer is simple, my blood-sugar averages are now down where they should be. My A1C test on November 7, 2010, had a reading of 6.9 (previously, it had been 13.3). The starting date of my work to correct the dawn effect and emergency glucose add was in May 2010. The bleeding in my eyes has fully healed, and my eyes look great. The eye doctor and retina specialist are ecstatic about my improvements. I have removed Actos from my pill lineup altogether. My lungs and kidneys have healed.

The massive water buildup in my legs and lower abdomen stopped. The legs have stopped weeping water and look way better. Early on, before we got the BG numbers and process cleaned up, I had a scrotum like a huge cannon ball between my legs. Specialists refused to help me until my doctor worked out where all the water was coming from, and a CAT scan confirmed it. (My body was adding water in an attempt to dilute all the glucose being dumped in by my liver. I did not want to become a maraschino cherry.)

By logging these numbers and working with my doctor, I got this monster under control. I have learned that my huge liver cannot be trusted to do the dawn effect, the Somogyi effect, and emergency glucose add. But I've cut off the dawn effect in its tracks with two metformin pills at 10:00 p.m. and 12:00 a.m.. I do not take both pills at once; that does not work for people like me. Metformin ER (extended release) pills are unreliable; I have tried them. To control the Somogyi sugar add takes watching the blood sugar so it does not go too low, adding glucose tablets and snacks as needed, and not instigating this mess. In the event you do end up with this mess, keep a wood pile and ax, an exercise machine, or good running shoes so you can exercise and blow off excess sugar as best you can.

It is ironic. I now spend more time ensuring my blood sugar does not go too low rather than too high. After February 2011 and the insulin change from Humalog 75/25 to Humalog Lispro standard insulin for all meals and no starlix pills, excessive lows and fast moving BG levels were no longer a problem.

# Chapter 5

# Continuous Glucose Monitor System (CGMS)

In January 2011, I obtained a Continuous Glucose Monitor System from Dexcom. I was unprepared for the impact of such technology. This system provides continuous monitoring of one's body glucose and displays it at any time on a small, handheld unit that one keeps close, within five feet.

The upshot was that I learned I was on the wrong insulin. My body was being driven from rail to rail on twelve-hour, strong, fast-acting 75/25 insulin on one side, although on the other side, the pancreas was really driving significant insulin on its own. The Starlix pills were too strong and were creating too much insulin.

Once I stopped taking the Starlix pills and started using needle-injected insulin for meals, the waveforms of my BG became far more stable and changed gently, and as stated earlier—like the waves on a placid lake. I added Humalog Lispro insulin at 5:30 am for startup and breakfast meal and for lunch and dinner as needed after meal  when my BG peaked above 180. This short duration insulin of five-hour duration and method of adding insulin as needed after lunch and dinner  also took the meal-eating schedule out of the medicines' hands and left it to me to schedule. Talk about relief.

Access to real-time data also allowed me to follow the timing and occurrence of unwarranted liver dumps when my BG was dropping or note when a slight bump occurred due to food-processing irregularities in my gut. These were stopped by taking metformin pills one hour before eating; ensuring that the metformin was up to strength in my blood prior to the fall off of the glucose output from the gut stopping sympathetic unwarranted liver dumps.

The more important issue is who needs or should use a CGMS.

Type 1 diabetic on insulin: this is a no brainer; you need a CGMS. If you are technical type, you too should have the latest in gizmos with a glucose gas gauge on your starship *Enterprise* front panel.

Anybody who does more than four finger sticks in a day to track his or her BG probably needs a CGMS. I was up to twenty to thirty-two sticks, chasing my monster, and needed a better picture. As I am now on full insulin, that closes the loop and question. If you cannot get a handle on your BG quickly and easily on four finger sticks a day, I recommend a CGMS for you.

Unfortunately, the technology is in its infancy. The computer-data logging aspects are old hat from the early days of industrial process control. The microminiaturization, radio links, and electronic wire sensors—which last three to seven days—are all new. My biggest beef is with the sensor technology, because replacing it and getting the next one to work appears to be a hit-and-miss situation, with the industry arguing about where to place the sensor—gut, butt, or upper arm. I had no success with the gut and always received the best response on the upper arm. A number of times a new sensor would work poorly and not track, and I'd have to place another one very carefully.

My most important advice is do not throw out your standard, handheld, finger-stick machine. You will need that to keep an eye on and calibrate the CGMS. Hopefully, you can get away with four or fewer strips a day. I usually have ten or more in case of a crisis when the sensor is not tracking properly.

# Chapter 6

## Pills

Folks, this chapter discusses key issues about pills and their impact on you. How long do your pills take to ingest and get to full strength? Once at full strength, how long do they last? At the end of a cycle, how long does it take for the pills to clear your body and be gone; is it a slow trickle or like the Niagara Falls?

Funny enough, nobody tells you to check this data; on top of that, you need to have idea about how these drugs work. Pills have basic functions and side effects that are all interacting with your body. As a diabetic, you need to get the available data, and measure these ingest times and up-to-strength times in the blood with a blood-glucose meter and a blood-pressure monitor.

Getting this data from your doctor or pharmacist can be real tricky. The Internet may be the best place to start your research on sites like Diabetes Self Management and Diabetes Forecast site. Originally, I had the mistaken belief that there was no such thing as an all-day pill. Then I ran into the glyburide insulin-generating pill that lasts ten hours. The classic "here, take one pill, and call me back in the morning" misses some extremely important facts. There you are, swallowing a pill as requested; it seems one a day is all you need, so you have been told; and yet there is a dirty dark secret: the left-out facts.

Five years ago, I was checking my blood pressure, curious about how the medicine was working, so I checked every hour, from early in the morning till late at night. I did that for a week, and imagine my horror when I found that it took two to three hours after swallowing the pill to see my blood pressure come down. It remained under control for four hours, and then after one hour, my blood pressure crawled back out to 180 over 115. Hey, wait a minute; those pills were supposed to be one a day and good all day. After calling the drug manufacturer, I learned that was not so; in fact, my data matched their worst drug-effigy case for intake (getting up to strength in the blood stream), effectiveness in the blood, and exit time. I am six feet, two inches tall and three hundred pounds, yes, overweight, but one-a-day pills are a crock no matter what your size is. The drug company safety officer told me to take more pills up front or a larger dose. I do not know what school these mutts went to. Adding larger doses or extra pills at front only ensures a stronger dose in blood and the same old  to live time of the pill. You can make a building taller by adding more pills on dose up front, but you cannot expand the base of building by doing that trick. Apparently some folks are super-blessed in that the pill effectiveness in their blood lasts a long time. But I have found that taking more doses spread over time is the only way to succeed for extended waking time coverage. At least, that is the case for me.

I do not have any use for the big bang theory of pill taking. The body does not redistribute the pill intake over a longer time frame but stuffs in more during the same interval. When I pushed the safety officer over this and said that I did not want to hammer my body with excess doses, he said I should redistribute and repeat the original small dose, spaced across twenty-four hours. After doing that, I had great blood-pressure readings all day.

I have a huge liver and big kidneys, and I reliably see my body strip pills out after intake and leave my body in a half-hour, like water flows over the Niagara Falls. I used to take the twenty-four-hour, big, white-bomber, delayed-response Claritin with Sudafed and was lucky if I got five to six hours of coverage. I got a similar response from my metformin pills. Originally, my doctor suggested taking one 1,000 mg pill in morning. I didn't feel good doing that so my doctor suggested splitting pill in half: 500 mg in morning and 500 mg at night. Later on, after testing the Accupril heart medicine and spinning it around the clock in small doses, the same to-live-time issue showed up with the metformin. It had a three-hour intake with a two-hour to-live time. Data from manufacturer suggested the to-live time was one to three hours. This layman saw two hours. Thus, I ended up with 500 mg doses spaced at 5:00 a.m., 12:00 p.m., and 7:00 p.m., after dinner. (Originally, before the extra midnight doses of metformin, the times were 8:00 a.m., 12:00 p.m., and 5:00 p.m.)

Later, my doctor decided to add two more 500 mg doses, one at 10:00 p.m. and one at midnight, which effectively cut off the dawn effect from 12:30 a.m. to 5:00 a.m. cutting off any extra glucose from liver. Even more interesting, the midnight dose did not add to the 10:00 p.m. dose already in the blood. In fact, it suffered the same ingestion delay and then dropped behind the 10:00 p.m. charge in the blood at the correct time; the to-live time of both doses was four hours at strength. Even more damning was that taking one large pill at 10:00 p.m. did not work. The liver was let out of its cage at 3:00 a.m. with a 1,000 mg dosage running around the blood system with a two-hour to-live time.

Never was so much time wasted by pill jockeys (not my excellent doctor) recommending that patients take one big, combined load. Crap. If you need an even dose over longer periods of time, this person learned without exception to take small, required doses around the clock as necessary. This has always worked well and correctly for me.

I did try some metformin ER pills that were supposed to have twice the time to live as standard metformin. Oh, hallelujah. Not so fast; after three days on these dogs—seeing my blood sugar readings all over the map and my dawn effect no longer properly cut off—I immediately switched back to standard metformin pills, and my benefits returned. As for the ER pills, it is not clear whether they were defective or could not be evenly digested. Medical advice of my Dr. Fung suggests that these modern, delayed-release pills do not work well in all people.

Metformin, in my mind, is a real miracle worker. I do not understand all that it does, but the trimming back of the liver's dawn effect is truly amazing. My layman's opinion is that whenever 500 mg metformin doses get up to strength in the blood stream, the liver cannot release blood glucose during this time. I also found that 250 mg doses will not do it. Also, the liver only stops releasing glucose when metformin is in the blood stream. There is no lasting effect from the drug after the to-live time in the blood starts winding down. In fact, between 5:30 a.m. and 6:00 a.m. and after the end of the midnight dose, and eating nothing, I can see the liver trying to make up for lost time when shutdown by metformin and then releasing more glucose to the blood stream, which keeps the BG rising. According to the Salk Institute:

Scientists discovered a genetic "fasting switch," called CRTC2, that flips on glucose production in the liver—the same switch that remains permanently on in patients with type II diabetes. A collaborative study among Salk researchers revealed that a common diabetes drug (metformin) works to inactivate CRTC2 and shut down glucose production. Having identified a molecular target for this drug, new, more active drugs will be easier to develop.

In healthy people, a "fasting switch" only flips on glucose production when blood glucose levels run low during fasting. "The existence of a second cellular signaling cascade—like an alternate route from A to B—that can modulate glucose production, presents the potential to identify new classes of drugs that might help to lower blood sugar by disrupting this alternative pathway,"

I found this information on the John Hopkins website:

Metformin, introduced as frontline therapy for uncomplicated Type 2 diabetes in the 1950s, up until now was believed to work by making the liver more sensitive to insulin. The Hopkins study shows, however, that metformin bypasses the stumbling block in communication and works directly in the liver cells.

Senior investigator Fred Wondisford MD, who heads the metabolism division at Hopkins Children's, tells us that, "Rather than an interpreter of insulin-liver communication, metformin takes over as the messenger itself. . . . Metformin actually mimics the action of CBP, the critical signaling protein involved in the communication between the liver and the pancreas that's necessary for maintaining glucose production by the liver and its suppression by insulin."

Regarding pills that enhance insulin production by the pancreas, prior to the full insulin approach, I was on glyburide and decided to return to the Starlix pills I'd been taking in the past. Despite my complaints about one-a-day pills, a glyburide pill does last ten hours.

This means depending upon how much insulin your pancreas is pushed to produce and how much glucose gets generated from the food you've eaten, you can have fun watching your blood sugar for ten hours. Once I was on full insulin with a five-hour maximum duration, that issue went away.

For someone who needs to prevent his BG from going too low and causing underruns, this aspect of a ten-and-a-half-hour glyburide and twelve-hour insulin is most unsavory and can really burn up the test strips in a day. Starlix is known as a fast-attack, short-strike pill that is organized around a meal. In a three-meal day—breakfast, lunch, and dinner (snacks excluded)—one could take three pills a day. I also have the option of dropping a pill in those cases when I need to miss a meal or reduce the pressure on my blood sugar. When using Starlix or glyburide, I have to eat sufficiently or there will be underruns. When taking liquid insulin on a all needle insulin stragtegy on Humalog Lispro on small doses  at each meal, I have the choice of adjusting the quantity of insulin to the food eaten. In a trying-to-lose-weight environment, an all liquid needle insulin approach  provides easier and better control.

Many times, when I was on the pills, prior to using liquid insulin, I would skip my lunchtime Starlix pill so I could snooze a couple of hours in the afternoon without fear of an emergency glucose dump. The Starlix pill provides much better flexibility than glyburide. As one is supposed to take Starlix at mealtime and not precede the meal by more than thirty minutes, Starlix and the digested sugars that are released are well coordinated and do not starve out the blood glucose supply. Typically, the pill lasts four hours, and if the glucose-generated meal is small, the body may have some spare insulin that requires a snack or glucose tablets.

When I used glyburide, given its long, active strength, it would burn off any extra glucose from my liver and gut late at night, after 9:00 p.m., and get my blood glucose down. Due to its four-hour cycle, Starlix was problematic on this issue as its extra insulin usually disappeared after 9:00 p.m. When I started with the liquid insulin, this issue was easily solved by an extra, small injection late at night. (In my body, the digestion process that converted fat to sugars was always completed six hours after I ate. This meant that if I ate dinner at 5:00 p.m., there would be a bump of the BG at 11:00 p.m.)

In summary, one-a-day pills and single – once daily large dose of 75/25 Insulin dose do not bear fruit for me. It is wise to check one's actual pill coverage. In case of the glyburide pill that does—contrary to all my experience—last ten hours, this is far more pain than it's worth. I'd have to eat all the time to keep it fed. At least with Starlix, I can skip a meal and omit the corresponding Starlix dose without grief. On liquid insulin, I simply add doses as necessary and to meet the glucose generated by a meal.

You really need to know your average digestion times, pill-intake time, and the length of time your insulin-hormone and metformin pills live in your blood so you can schedule things and do not have to monitor your blood-sugar levels every fifteen minutes. The tighter you try to run your diet to lose weight, the more you will need to watch the factors I've mentioned here, as there will be times when low or no glucose will come out of your gut or liver to work on any extra insulin floating around. Remember that anything you do must be under your doctor's care and express approval.

On a side note, carefully watch and check your other prescriptions—antibiotics, etc. Check carefully for anything that will interact with your diabetic medicines; such complications may cause surprise hyperglycemic or hypoglycemic events. This is not a trivial matter. One drug class to watch like a hawk is Levaquin and its related drugs. In my case, this drug overrode my metformin and caused the liver to secrete all sorts of glucose andraise my BG continuously and gradually increase it until it was over 232 on an empty stomach. In addition, I had to use twice as much insulin. After one day I stopped taking it, and my blood glucose levels returned back to normal.

Finally, what a change a year makes. I exercised hard, controlled my diet, and added the CGMS. In April 2011, I yanked the Starlix out, changed the insulin type, and revised my doses dramatically. For safety's sake, it is best to be on a CGMS when making such changes.

# Chapter 7

## Medicine List and Recipe

The first list is a result of all the data I've obtained from the CGMS. For comparison, I have also included my prior, pre-CGMS list as things were working in a fashion at that time. Then in February 2011, things changed dramatically while I was on the CGMS. These lists itemize my medications as they pertain to my type 2 diabetes. I also take high-blood-pressure pills, 325 mg of aspirin daily, diuretics, and asthma treatments but have left them off for clarity. They do not have a significant impact on type 2 diabetes, as best as I can tell.

The list reflects the change in insulin type from 23 units of Humalog 75/25 once a day to four shots a day of Humalog Lispro, where each shot is one-half to four units. In addition, to cut out liver dumps after the gut-and-liver digestion completion and falling output, I retimed the metformin and related pills to one hour before starting a meal so that the up-to-strength time of the metformin in the blood system (a two-and-a-half-hour delay) beats the gut completion and resulting falling BG and prevents errant liver dumps. My gut's usual completion delay is usually one and a half to two hours with normal meals.

The Humalog Lispro dose was usually four units for breakfast, three units for lunch, three units for dinner, and a half dose at 11:00 p.m. to help keep the wee hours quiet and stable.

I varied my dose injection times in a special way. The breakfast dose was taken at 5:30 a.m. to help catch the liver attempting to do dawn affect after being shutdown due to the midnight 500 mg metformin dose. That metformin dose usually wears off at 5:30 a.m., and the BG starts climbing.I also found that my body, after thirty years on other regimens, in fact was working better than had been anticipated. After I removed the large dose of Humalog 75/25 and the 12-hour-duration insulin in the morning, the CGMS began recording BG drops every time I started eating. That indicated that the stomach was properly signaling the pancreas to release the meal bolus or bulk release. As a result, the lunch and dinner doses and the optional extra dose after breakfast were determined by watching after meal completion; how far the BG peaked up as blood glucose would be absorbed at the behest of available released insulin. I would usually add a three-unit dose when the BG climbed to 190 or higher. Taking it any sooner would add to the pancreas meal bolus at the start of the meal and ran risk of lowering BG too much. Tacked on the end, it helped suppress the peak and as long as it was not too large, it would not crash the BG when my gut emptied.

I tried to take the lunch dose no later than 1:30 p.m. and the dinner dose no later than 6:30 p.m. Humalog Lispro has five-hour lasting time, which covers the hours from 1:30 p.m. to 6:30 p.m. and 6:30 p.m. to 11:30 p.m. Finally, I also added a half—to one-unit dose at 11:30 p.m. to help me get through the night.

These approaches helped get the BG to be more like the waves on a placid lake and stop the massive cycling and swinging, and save test strips and make glucose tablets unnecessary.

My latest recipe on the CGMS is as follows:

5:00 a.m. Take a wake-up reading of my BG on my left hand and right hand. Have small, one hundred-calorie snack of nuts and cheese.

5:30 a.m. Take a four-unit dose of Humalog Lispro. In my case, if I'd had an emergency sugar add the day before, I usually find that the liver has dumped all of its spare glucose the night before and has nothing to add in its attempt to do the dawn effect at 5:30 a.m. As a result, the morning Humalog will have little to do.

6:15 a.m. 500 mg of metformin. Take vitamins and other medicine.

6:30–7:00 a.m. Eat breakfast.

7:45 a.m. Walk quarter-mile loops around condo park. Check BG after every loop to be sure not to bottom out. I stop when the BG hits 140. I always wait a minimum of thirty minutes after eating so I do not rush the contents of the stomach into the intestines.

9:00 a.m. Typically, I see the gut start to empty between 9:00 and 9:30 a.m. The metformin I've taken earlier gets up to strength around 8:45 a.m. and is ready to block any liver dump that may occur. I always check to see how high the BG is peaking; and if it is over 180, I add one and a half to two shots of Humalog Lispro and carefully note and log the time. It lasts five hours.

11:00 a.m. 500 mg of metformin, heart pills, diuretic.

12:00–12:30 p.m. Lunch. The metformin is synced to the lunchtime meal.

1:00–3:30 p.m. Watch the CGMS trend line, and when the BG peaks over 180 to 190, inject three units of Humalog Lispro, no later than 1:30 p.m. If the BG stays under 180, I do not take an injection. My gut usually runs out within one and a half to two and a half hours. An early metformin pill with the noon meal usually means that it gets up to strength by 1:30 p.m., beating the gut's completion of digestion and preventing a liver dump as the BG heads back down. 4:00 p.m. 500 mg of metformin and Accupril pills.

5:00–6:00 p.m. Typically, I have my dinner at this time. Any later stretches out the digestion time at night, making it hard to get the BG back under 140. The metformin is synced to the dinner meal.

5:00–6:30 p.m. Watch the CGMS trend line, and when the BG peaks over 180 to 190, inject three units of Humalog Lispro, no later than 6:30 p.m. If the BG stays under 180, I do not take an injection. My gut usually runs out in one and a half to two and a half hours. A metformin pill at 4:00 p.m. usually means it is up to strength by 6:30 p.m., beating the gut's completion of digestion and preventing a liver dump as the BG heads back down as gut empties.

9:30 p.m. Lantus shot; 15 units always. Adjust the quantity based on the slope of line on the CGMS graph over the midnight hours. Lantus is a basal insulin that lasts twenty-four hours and supposedly has no peaks like Humalog.

10:00 p.m. 500 mg metformin pill to shut down the dawn effect from 12:30 a.m. to 3:00 a.m.

12:00 a.m. 500 mg metformin pill to shut down the dawn effect from 3:00 a.m. to 5:30 a.m.

In summary, my sense of all this was:

- 75/25 Humalog Insulin that lasts twelve hours and glyburide pills that last ten and a half hours are a right pain in the butt, causing one to eat constantly.
- Starlix is no longer necessary and was a heavy hammer. Now insulin injections of the correct type facilitate simpler and better control, and meal times can be more flexible.
- The CGMS allows a safer, tighter, and simplified control approach, as shown here, and minimizes the insulin used to a bare minimum.
- A short-acting—five hour duration—insulin such as Humalog Lispro provides an easier control approach and facilitates weight loss without excess pressure from the twelve-hour insulin.
- Timing the metformin doses is crucial to stopping inappropriate liver dumps after the gut empties out and the BG starts to dip as gut empties and BG sometimes bounce up and down due to more food trailing after meal digestion (not due to low BG either). Eating a new snack shortly after eating main meal can cause this effect.

My previous, pre-CGMS pill list (until February 2011):

5:00 a.m. 500 mg of metformin and 23 units of Humalog 75/25. Take wake-up reading of BG, vitamins, and other medicine (one hour after the Humalog injection). If I'd had an emergency sugar add the day before, I usually find that the liver/brain has dumped all of its spare glucose night before and has nothing to add in its attempt to do the dawn effect at 5:30 a.m. As a result, my morning Humalog dose will have little to do and may need reduction of dose.

6:00 a.m. Have a small, fifty-calorie snack—a piece of ham and a small amount of carbohydrates.

6:30 a.m. Walk quarter-mile loops of condo park. Check BG after every loop to be sure not to bottom out. I stop at 140.

8:00 a.m. Ingest Starlix pill. Eat breakfast. If there is too much insulin pressure from the Humalog and the breakfast Starlix, I drop the breakfast Starlix and let the Humalog do all the work till lunch.9:00 a.m. Check my BG to ensure that the gut is outputting sugar 140 to 180. The Starlix pill and the resulting insulin created should hold the BG around 140 to 170, assuming I have not exceeded my diet. If I get 190 to 200-plus, I immediately go for a quarter-mile walk to wear off the excess glucose and get it back to 170 or less.

10:00 a.m. Typically my BG starts to drop around 10:00 a.m., indicating that the gut is running down on its input. If so, I add a small snack to help cover the insulin till 12:00 p.m., when the Starlix will run out after its four-hour cycle. I skip the snack if the BG holds to 170 or more through 11:00 a.m. I will have eaten enough to ensure a full four hours of insulin production. I really want a little excess of unoccupied insulin near the end of the Starlix/insulin period to help drive the BG back to 110 to 140. If there is no spare insulin left from the Starlix/pancreas action, it means I've either eaten too much or the wrong foods or both.

12:00–1:00 p.m. 500 mg of metformin, heart pills, diuretic. Have lunch; take Starlix pill, which is synced to the lunchtime meal. (If I skip lunch, I do not take the Starlix.)

1:15 p.m. Check BG to ensure the gut is outputting sugar 140 to 180. The Starlix pill and the insulin created as a result should hold the BG at 140 to 170, assuming I have not exceeded my diet. If it gets to 190 to 200-plus, I immediately go for a quarter-mile walk to wear off excess glucose and get it back to 170 to 180.

3:00 p.m. Typically, my BG starts to drop around 3:00 p.m. or earlier, an indication that the gut is decreasing its input. If so, I add a small snack to help cover the insulin till 5:00 p.m. when the Starlix will run out after its four-hour cycle. I will skip the snack if the BG holds to 170 or more between 2:30 and 5:00 p.m. as that indicates I have eaten enough to ensure a full four hours of insulin production. Usually, I want to have a little excess of unoccupied insulin near the end of the Starlix/insulin period to help drive the BG back to 110 to 140. If there is no spare insulin left after the Starlix/pancreas action, that means I have either eaten too much or the wrong foods (or both). Breakfast and dinner usually occupy most of the four-hour Starlix period with lunch being shortest period. At least, that's how it was for me, and I was always struggling from the glucose running out and having to eat extra snacks.

5:00–6:00 p.m. Eat dinner. Eating any later that this always stretched out the digestion time at night, making it hard to get my BG back under 140. Take Starlix pill. If I skip dinner, I do not take the pill. As mentioned above, the Starlix is synced to the evening meal.6:15 p.m. Check the BG to ensure my gut is outputting sugar 140 to 180. The Starlix pill and the insulin created as a result should hold the BG to 140 to 170, assuming I have not exceeded my diet. If it is 190 to 200-plus, I immediately go for a quarter-mile walk to wear off the excess glucose and get it back to 170 to 180.

8:30–9:00 p.m. Typically I see my BG start to drop around 8:45 p.m., which indicates that my gut is decreasing its output of glucose. I will not add a snack at this point; at most, I will take some glucose tablets or part of one, if my blood glucose gets too low. After taking the dinnertime Starlix, I usually see that dinner digestion does not end too early. My sugar usually is 150 to 160 at the end of the Starlix four-hour period. Usually the strong output from the gut usually lasts till 9:00 p.m., and the BG drops as my gut and liver cannot keep up such a strong output. There are still remnants being digested slowly from 9:00 p.m. to midnight. These last amounts of glucose cause the BG numbers to crawl up to 180. Typically, at the end of a Starlix period, I may see my BG jump from the 130s to the 160s as a result of the last, slow output from my liver and gut.

9:30 p.m. Fifteen units of Lantus, shot at one time.

Balance of pill schedule and items left out of meal discussion::

7:00 p.m. 500 mg of metformin and a blood-pressure pill, Accupril. This is taken here because the metformin will be active in the blood from 10:00 p.m. through 12:00 a.m., stopping the liver's glucose production and leakage and making it easier to get my BG numbers low and stabilized before I go to bed at midnight.

10:00 p.m. 500 mg of metformin to shut down the dawn effect between 12:30 a.m. and 3:00 a.m.

12:00 a.m. 500 mg of metformin to shut down the dawn effect between 3:00 a.m. and 5:30 a.m.

In summary, my sense of all this was that:

- From the morning to lunch, all was well and straightforward.
- It was always wise to check my BG between 10:15 and 10:45 a.m. to guard against the Humalog's peak release of its slow insulin.
- The afternoon was always a riot, trying to get in a snack around 2:30 to 5:00 p.m.
- No snacks two and a half hours before my next meal.
- Once I ingest a Starlix pill, I am committed to eat within that four-hour period and ensuring that the insulin created by the pill's action on the pancreas is loaded. To skip a meal, I also had to skip the corresponding Starlix pill, otherwise I'd have to reach for glucose tablets and snacks, without exception.
- Lastly, earlier when I could not lose any of my excess weight, I had configured my diet to twelve hundred calories gross and fifteen hundred calories net. This added extra pressure because the insulin was always a little unloaded. I needed to keep up very active BG-meter checking to catch underruns and add snacks and glucose tablets where needed. Increasing calories will reduce that pressure.
- Due to excess pressure of 75/25 Humalog insulin in am meant I had to keep BG above 140 and preferably around 160 to 180 when doing any activities to prevent the BG descending straight down to sub 100. Under this 75/25 Insulin; my BG when it got to 110 would descend to 54 and cause a emergency liver dump sending my Blood Glucose BG to 278. Doctor's order was to keep BG above 100 at all times. Once on the latest Meds list on CGMS with standard Humalog Lispro Insulin in smaller doses and no Starlix this was no longer an issue.

I developed the following chart to help me keep track of my medications (revised February 28, 2011———CGMS.)

| TIME/ ACTIVITY | QTY | DESCRIPTION | TYPE | DOSE | REASON |
|---|---|---|---|---|---|
| 5:00 a.m. Wake up | | | | Take morning finger sticks. | |
| | 100 Cal | Snack | | Low-glycemic load | |
| 5:30 a.m. | 4 | Humalog Lispro | Needle | IU | Diabetes insulin |
| 6:15 a.m. | ½ | Metformin | Tablet | 1,000 mg | Basic treatment for diabetes |
| | | Vitamin supplements | | As detailed | |
| | 1 | Furosemide | Tablet | 20 mg | Tissue swelling |
| 6:30 a.m. Breakfast | | | 300-calorie, low-glycemic diet | | |
| Check BG if GT is 180 | 3 | Humalog Lispro | Needle | IU | Use CGMS and add insulin if peak is too high. |
| 11:00 a.m. | ½ | Metformin | Tablet | 1,000 mg | |
| | 1 | Furosemide | Tablet | 20 mg | |
| 12:00 p.m. Lunch | | | | | |
| Check BG if GT 180 | 3 | Humalog Lispro | Needle | IU | Diabetes Insulin – take by 1:30 p.m. |
| 4:00 p.m. | ½ | Metformin | Tablet | 1,000 mg | |
| 5:00 p.m. | | | | | |

| Dinner | | | | | |
|---|---|---|---|---|---|
| Check BG if GT 180 | 3 | Humalog Lispro | Needle | IU | Diabetes insulin; take by 6:30 p.m. |
| 9:30 p.m. | 15 | Lantus | Needle | IU | Diabetes basil insulin shot |
| 10:00 p.m. | ½ | Metformin | Tablet | 1,000 MG | |
| 11:30 p.m | .½ to 1 | Humalog Lispro | Needle | IU | Keeps BG down at night. |
| 12:00 a.m. | ½ | Metformin | Tablet | 1,000 mg | |

# Chapter 8

# Daily Routine: Summary and Overview

This chapter may seem like a duplication of prior chapters, but its role is to summarize the key events and objectives and the "why" about what is going on.

My daily routine starts at 5:00 a.m., when my alarm clock rings. I wake up and immediately measure my blood sugar. I want it to be 140 and below if possible, but it can range up to 180.

If the dawn effect has not been stopped by the 10:00 p.m. and 12:00 a.m. metformin pills, this number will be high, around 238 to 245 or higher. I take a low-glycemic, 100-calorie snack of nuts.

I take four units of Humalog Lispro at 5:30 a.m.I take the next metformin pill of 500 mg at 6:15 a.m., along with my vitamin supplements.

I eat a breakfast of 300 calories between 6:30 and 7:00 a.m.

I walk at 7:30 a.m. for exercise.By 8:45, the 6:15 a.m. metformin dose is now strong enough in the blood system to stop the liver glucose release and shut down the dawn effect. I call that re-caging the liver. The insulin shot at 5:30 a.m. also helps to stop the effect.

I take a 500 mg metformin pill plus heart pills at 11:00 a.m. followed by lunch between 12:00 and 12:30 p.m.

I monitor my BG between 12:30 and 3:30 p.m. to catch the peak on the CGMS. Once the CGMS shows that my BG has peaked over 180 and it is no later than 1:30 p.m., I add three units of insulin. If the BG continues up above 190, I add another four units. If the BG does not exceed 180, I do not add any insulin.

I take a 500 mg metformin pill and heart pills at 4:00 p.m. followed by dinner from 5:00 to 6:00 p.m.

I monitor my BG between 5:30 and 9:30 p.m. to catch the peak on the CGMS. Once the BG peaks over 180 and if it is no later than 6:30 p.m., I add three units of insulin. If the BG continues up above 190, I add another four units. If the BG does not exceed 180, I do not add any insulin.

I do not eat any snack after dinner or drink any fluids that need active digestion as I find that the heavy part of digestion is usually over in four hours, by 9:00 to 10:00 p.m. This is desirable so that the 6:30 Dinner Insulin shot covers the meal so that the evening BG will be drawn down..

At 9:30 p.m., I take single shot of 15 units of Lantus, which works fine.

My goal is to have the BG as low as I can get—to 140 or lower—when I sleep. That's why there are no more snacks—"mid-rats"—navy for "midnight rations"—after dinner is done.

To help keep the midnight BG down, I take one-half to one unit of insulin at 11:30 p.m. Note: I usually find that six hours after eating a meal, I will see one more dump of glucose from the fat digestion, and then gut will remains empty and calm.

At 10:00 p.m. and midnight, I take a dose of metformin. This is based upon my body's tendency to take two and a half hours to go from ingest to strength, spend two hours at strength, and half an hour to leave. Most metformin pills work okay, but I have issues with metformin ER. This gives me uninterrupted coverage and blocks the dawn effect from 12:30 a.m. through 5:30 a.m.

# Chapter 9

## Diet and Other Rain Dances

Folks, diets and which one to follow—low fat/some fat, low glycemic versus high glycemic, etc.—present a minefield of important issues, approaches, and contending philosophies. There truly is a contrast from the young growing person who has an ability to eat any and lots of interesting foods and the older person who simply does not need tons of energy to keep rolling.

It's like the story of the pharaohs in Egypt. If you are moving two-ton stone blocks for the pharaoh's tombs and edifices, you'd better eat the best lowland carbohydrates the Nile can produce. If you are only watching and supervising the construction, you'd better be on a low-carbohydrate diet. Mummies that have been examined clearly show the problems—diabetes, etc.—the pharaohs experienced. No matter which diet/approach you end up using, the diet you follow must provide sufficient carbohydrates/calories to keep your body functioning without overwhelming your body and rotting out your whole body from excess glucose as well as providing necessary nutrients, vitamins, fiber etc to keep your body functioning correctly without excessive weight gain.

One of the problems many of us face is that, genetically, our bodies are intended to be on the old hunter-gatherer diet: chicken, fish, nuts, vegetables, fruits, etc. Highly refined carbohydrates are not part of that list. Carbohydrates—bread, cakes, cereals, buns, pasta, potatoes, rice, cereal, grains, etc.—are converted into glucose

37

in the body. In fact, you can count carbohydrates to estimate how much glucose will hit your blood system. Remember that the body needs some carbohydrates just to keep rolling. If you go all low glycemic, you can end up starving your body of glucose. The liver will be forced to add glucose, and you'll hope your BG will remain under control without blowing up your blood-sugar averages.

I follow the recommendations that suggest carbohydrates should only be 20 percent of one's diet. Typical dinner would consist of: arger portions of green vegetables, six-ounce portions of meat, etc., and fresh fruit. I like the Mediterranean diet as well: two glasses a day of dark red wine for men and one for women. Most of this data came from the Diabetes Self Management website and blogs. www.diabetesselfmanagement.com; www.tudiabetes.org; www.forecast.diabetes.org (ADA); heatlthcarecenter@womentowomen.com

I have organized my diet to have a target of thirteen hundred calories gross: two hundred fifty for breakfast, two hundred fifty for lunch, seven hundred for dinner, and one hundred for snacks. I started doing this as I was grossly overweight, and I am now working it down. I may slide to fifteen hundred calories net by the end of day. As I am now on a full insulin regimen and no oral pills like starlix or glyburide, I load insulin as needed by watching the CGMS to see when the BG peaks. If you are on pills such as Starlix or glyburide and trying to lose weight, you need to ensure that you are eating sufficient carbohydrates and food to keep the pills occupied or you will have hypoglycemic, low-BG periods. You'll have to test more, watch out for the glucose starve out at the end of a meal, and add a glucose tablet or snacks to prevent the liver and brain from doing an emergency glucose add. When I was on Starlix pills, failure to eat sufficient food forced my liver to ram my blood glucose to 275 and higher.

My diet may seem somewhat lean, but I want my blood sugar always coming down. When I was on Starlix and glyburide pills, I added snacks at 9:30 and 1:30 p.m. This was not needed when I began taking full insulin using needles throughout the day and not just the one shot in the early morning of 75/25 insulin and oral pills—Starlix at every meal.

This section is meant to be a thumbnail sketch; there are excellent websites and self-help resources such as Diabetes Self Management website available with more information on diets. If you live alone, implementing this diet will not be problematic. If you live with another person, who maybe does all the cooking or shares that task with you, chances are the other party is not diabetic; if he or she eats with you, he or she will always be hungry and feel starved. Varying one's routine always invites errors and can create riots within your friends and family.

Even low-glycemic food in portions that are too large will be a problem; for diabetics, portions should be baby sized. Then you have the battle of how many carbohydrates to take. Too much, and your blood sugar goes through the roof; not enough, and you get an early burn out of carbohydrates and if you are not watching, your liver will be forced to add glucose. When using needle-injected insulin, one counts and estimates carbohydrates to match the meal; if one is on Starlix or glyburide pills, one needs to eat sufficient food and add extra snacks where necessary.

One very important aspect of this is timing. Are you on needle-injected insulin (and not twelve-hour-lasting insulin) or on Starlix or glyburide pills? If losing weight is a concern, twelve-hour-lasting insulin and ten-and-a-half-hour glyburide pills will drive your schedule, forcing you to eat to prevent lows. Starlix pills are slightly better than glyburide pills in that the former lasts four hours. Once you swallow the pill, though, you are committed to four hours of eating and digesting a meal. The thing to determine is, Are you scheduling your meals, or are your medicines scheduling you?

The twelve-hour-lasting insulin or glyburide pills make traveling and visiting with out-of-town friends and family challenging. Trying to hold meals to a hard schedule can be daunting. When I was on Starlix or glyburide pills, the best approach (so I could be flexible) was to substitute snacks for meals sometimes and switch out later snacks with full meals. With this approach, I could maintain other folks required schedules without blowing up my schedule. To reduce glucose overload from strange meals in restaurants and fast foods, I followed a low-glycemic approach: meat(typically chicken or fish), vegetables, and small serving of starches (a corner of a bun, four french fries, etc.) Oh yes, I'd remove fried flour coatings from chicken, etc.; otherwise there were no buns, bread, pasta, rice, or potatoes. Doing this turned out to be most helpful and allowed me to safely select items in restaurants. The other thing I did was run my blood sugar a little higher—170 to 180—while traveling to minimize underruns while I was standing in line for security at airports, shopping with friends, and visiting. During rest times, I'd walk around the hotel or stores to get my blood sugar lower during inactive, waiting times. This approach saved test strips and the opportunity for an under run on my blood sugar. Eating on my earlier regimen required a regular schedule, which is crucial in order to know when the low blood sugar points show up, which you can easily test and then eat a snack. Fifo buffer and emergency functions of liver could not be trusted. Liver not signaling on insulin properly and overloading glucose release to load just sufficient glucose. In the under run situation, this means that at one point my BG was at 70, and twenty minutes later, it would be at 265, blowing up all my averages, not to mention adding excess sugar to my organs. If your body is still working reasonably, this may not be issue yet.

Keep an eye on this periodically.My typical dinner would be six to eight ounces of fish or roasted chicken, eight or more ounces of green beans or mixed vegetables, and a quarter-cup of potatoes, rice, or pasta, etc., followed by dried or fresh fruit for dessert. I love beef, especially rib eye, prime rib, tri-tip, and steak. These types of beef, while delectable, are very rich, take longer to digest, and can easily throw off your numbers. Eat small portions, no more than six ounces.

One factor needing careful watching and observing is the digestion time of your body. For me, it is two to two and a half hours maximum until glucose shows up in numbers in blood. I do not eat snacks later than two and a half hours before my next meal so I do not preload my next meal.

In addition, when I was on the oral Starlix/glyburide, I needed to take the Starlix pill early enough (for me, this was ten to fifteen minutes) before the meal to prevent a huge bump in the BG before Starlix and pancreas can fire up the insulin. If you take it too early, you crater your BG level; too late, you get a huge bump. Later being on full insulin; this was no longer an issue.

I usually find that the sugars from fat digestion are always produced six hours after ingestion providing a bump of the BG level up to 180 to 190.

In summary, following a simple, good low-glycemic diet with sufficient but minimum carbohydrates will be super-critical to getting blood-sugar levels and your type 2 diabetes under control.

In the early phases of my disease before the metformin dawn effect fix, one of the key meals where I had to carefully choose foods and watch calories was breakfast. The problem has to do with the human body as it has been shut down all night while asleep. Insulin is very low, the liver had loaded up my body with excessive glucose, and on top of that, ingested pills would take up to two and a half to three hours ingestion to get back to functioning correctly.

On top of all that, any calories consumed for snack or breakfast would immediately hit my system and elevate the BG above 238. Due to the huge glucose add by the liver in early am, adding 26 units of 75/25 insulin had virtually no effect (due to insulin resistance) until after two hours of walking two miles to get the excess glucose unloaded.

The bottom line was that any snack/breakfast (forty-five to one hundred calories) had to be protein—low glycemic—to reduce BG boost from calories. By lunchtime, this was no longer a problem. In addition, once the metformin was used to shut down the dawn effect, the body worked more normally at wakeup, and the Humalog Lispro insulin worked immediately at wakeup without showing insulin resistance.

For me, insulin resistance is the effect of the body cells refusing to absorb any more glucose from the blood stream. Usually more insulin can overcome that but as it gets worse, drugs like Actos are required to force more glucose in. What I repeatedly found is that hearty exercise will force the glucose out of the cells so they can take more in and that is why hearty exercise is essential to good glucose control. If you are on oral pills such as metformin, Starlix, or glyburide or have strong insulin resistance, you will want to hold off two to three hours from eating any extra carbohydrates in the morning till the med's up to strength—full action- and the blood sugar is stabilized. This means a super-low-glycemic breakfast with a very small portion of carbohydrates. Forget about toast and cereals. As a result of this problem in the early phases of my diabetes, I ended up with a very low-glycemic breakfast and no breads, cereals, rice, etc. It was hard enough walking two miles at 6:00 a.m. each and every day without adding more glucose to the 235–65 starting point. Today with the dawn effect corralled and on a full insulin strategy and no oral Starlix/glyburide, I believe it is still appropriate to start with a very low-glycemic breakfast and ease the startup load of my body and sugars.

In addition, when on the early regimen, I would see more normal behavior by lunch, and the canned cream/Coffee-mate riot had not occurred. This sensitivity was hilarious one day when I was looking for a very low-sugar Coffee-mate. I found one that had no sugars added (except for the corn-syrup solids that are added as a base), and I drank my coffee and whee! Forty units up on blood sugar. The response I received from the manufacturer was priceless. They can advertise it that way as long as they also note the other sugars (even if in a non-obvious way with an asterisk and a tiny footnote on the bottle)

# Chapter 10

## Vitamins and Their Ilk

Given my age of sixty-two-plus, difficulties to date, and all the advice out there on the Web, in health blogs, and newspapers, it is good form and just a sane bet to take vitamins. Years back, it would be rare to catch me ingesting a single multivitamin.

Today, I take a handful of these babies, and so far no damage has occurred and my health has been improving. The list below is provided for interest; as previously indicated, be sure to check with your doctor prior to taking any new vitamins.

Here are the vitamins I take; unless noted otherwise, I take these now at 6:15 a.m.:

1. 900 mg of glucosamine and chondroitin, one per meal.
2. 400 mg of magnesium oxide, one per day.
3. 6 mg of lutein for my eyes, one per day.
4. 1,200 mg of fish oil, 600 mg total EPA and DHA, one per day.

Eicosapentaenoic acid – docosahexaenoic acid

5. 200 micrograms (mcg) chromium picolinate, one per day.
6. 5,000 IU vitamin D3, one per day.
7. 1,000 mcg vitamin B12, one per day.

Neuron growth factor (NGF), 320 mg acetyl L-carnitine arginate DiHCL, 300 mg acetyl L-carnitine HCL (VRC), two capsules in morning and night.

8. Cerovite Senior multivitamin or the equivalent, one per day.

9. 1,000 mg vitamin C ascorbic acid fine crystals (antioxidant), one dose per day.

10. Deep red wine such as merlot or ruby cabernet, two glasses per day for a man, one per day for a woman, morning and afternoon after meals. Improves the blood vessels in the brain.

# Chapter 11

## Booze and Having a Drink

Despite the chance I'll be tagged as a boozer and hellhound, I'll admit to liking a good drink of ethyl alcohol on an occasional basis. This is because I am originally from Canada, where having a good drink is right up there with manliness. Thus, this chapter is *not* a chapter on reformation and dropping bad habits; neither is it a request for all else to follow suit. My point here, however, is that if you are properly watching what you eat and do not want to bottom out your blood sugar, there are some key thoughts to keep in mind about alcohol.

I was quite shocked to learn critical data of the impact that alcohol has on the body. I am not talking about cirrhosis of the liver and other diseases that come from alcohol abuse. The engine of alcohol processing is the liver, which cannot process sugars/carbohydrates and alcohol at the same time. Alcohol always takes priority. It is also true that every cell in the body can process small amounts of ethyl alcohol, without the aid of insulin or glucose. The net effect is that if people with diabetes drink large quantities of wine or hard liquor, their livers will stop processing sugar until the liver is finished processing the alcohol. To prevent blood-glucose underruns, they may need to take glucose tablets. However, I generally find that an occasional glass of wine, sipped over a period of time, is not much of an issue. It's probably a good idea to carefully review our BG numbers and identify the best time to have a drink. When I'm using

Starlix, the best time is between doses, around lunch and before dinner. The least ideal time is right after an insulin shot or after taking Starlix or glyburide pills because then the extra sugar in the BG will be at its lightest, and the alcohol will have its worst impact. I also discovered that alcohol shuts down the beneficial effects of metformin on the liver resulting in excess liver glucose release. I then realized that the best time for me to have a drink—slow sips of wine—was when I woke up, when the gut is empty and there is no metformin rattling around my system. The simple answer is not to take both metformin and hard liquor at same time.

From a losing-weight perspective, alcohol adds calories and needs to be factored into your diet calculations. Otherwise enjoy an occasional drink of deep red wine to provide benefits to your body and brain. Be careful, as moderation is the key, and good luck.

# Chapter 12

## Exercise

Folks, there are many fine organizations—from outpatient groups at hospitals to professional gyms—that provide detailed and balanced programs to answer many rehabilitation and exercise needs.

It is absolutely critical for people with type 2 diabetes to do regular hearty exercise on a daily basis. Hearty regular exercise, maintaining your diet, and metering are the keys to better control of the disease. They all must be done without fail in conjunction with taking medicine. Regular hearty exercise is key to keeping insulin resistance down and glucose being consumed and removed from the blood stream, good weight control and body in good shape.

I found taking a quarter-mile walk around my condo park to be fine, and adding more loops can get this walk up to two or three miles. Another excellent exercise is to pick up a broom, shovel, or snow shovel, which is even more effective at burning off the calories. Two years ago, when I had elevated BG levels that would not drop below 180, exercise smoked out a solution. If I walked two miles every day, I could get the BG down to a 100 or less. I had a diet of twelve hundred calories that I still eat today, but back then I was losing no weight and in fact reached 330 pounds. Finally in May 2010, this problem was tracked to my liver and signaling systems: the dawn effect was dumping in glucose every morning, up to 238 to 258. An emergency glucose add during waking hours was doing similar stunts, overloading my body to 278. Adding 500 mg of metformin at 10:00 p.m. and 12:00 a.m. cut off that dawn affect until 5 a.m. With extensive metering, I was able to cut off the liver dump by preventing the blood glucose from getting under 100. Then my daily numbers and ranges were at the place they were supposed to be, and by November 7, 2010, my A1C was a respectable 6.9. To restate, this paragraph highlights the critical importance of hearty exercise and was instrumental in solving this poor glucose control and arriving at a solution.

A special note here about fast-acting, strong insulin: it can result in your BG moving and responding too quickly. When I was on Humalog 75/25 with a twelve-hour duration, I would see my BG move up and down so fast that a CGMS could not track the changes. Today, I am on a proper regimen of Humalog Lispro with small doses and duration of five hours, and this is no longer an issue.

One factor to remember is that your BG must be high enough to support exercise. When I was on the original Humalog 75/25 plus the Starlix and metformin pills, typically, a quarter-mile walk would subtract 11 to 16 units from the BG; when the insulin pressure was up, then 20 units could be knocked off. My later regimen on Humalog Lispro standard, five-hour insulin and metformin did not show these wild changes.

When I was using Humalog 75/25 12-hour insulin and Starlix pills, in order to prevent underruns and ensure I had sufficient BG, I would want my BG up at 180 when I exercised. Using the snow shovel, sweeping leaves, etc., watch out; with a body like mine, I could burn through my available blood glucose in fifteen minutes and had to check and load more fuel in the boiler if needed. As indicated, an insulin regimen and pill intake need careful review. For me, being on regular all insulin five-hour Humalog Lispro insulin, in smaller better doses, and metformin, these protective issues were not necessary. I raise these concerns as I had to live with them for four years, fighting this mess.

Be warned, under heavy exercise you will need lots of glucose, so closely monitor your BG levels, and add energy as needed. Once you are back in the house, sitting down or at computer, your fuel load (food—carbohydrates) will need to be reduced to the minimum again.

Typically, I walk one and a half to two miles each day to keep everything rolling properly. Today, anytime my BG increases above 180, I add three to four units of Humalog Lispro and also walk quarter-mile loops until the sugar gets below 180.

# Chapter 13

## Heartaches and Tears

I found the destruction of my prior life routines coupled with the lack of flexibility and the hard pill and meal schedules annoying, frustrating, depressing, and a nuisance. It took weeks, months to figure out the recipe—diet, pills, insulin shots, exercise, and schedule—until it became second nature and somewhat, as much as possible, of a daily routine with better-managed blood sugar numbers. Drug-enforced meal schedules caused by twelve-hour duration 75/25 insulin coupled with oral medications coupled with Starlix or glyburide and reduced eating amounts can drive one absolutely nuts. Once I was on an all-insulin needle strategy that had a five-hour duration with reduced doses and no oral Starlix/glyburide, life improved dramatically. My wife became totally frustrated over my diets and what to feed me. Simply stated, I needed to watch my grains, rice, potatoes, starchy food, pasta, and breads so I did not blow up my diet. That is the tricky and sometimes frustrating part. I realized I needed to have smaller meals and probably two snacks when on the 75/25 insulin plus starlix a day to level out the body's glucose supply. Being on an all needle insulin strategy also eliminated the extra snacks and daily use of glucose tablets eliminated.

When you are at home, following a diet and exercise routine can be relatively straightforward and provides the least risk of losing control. Vacations, going out with friends for dinner, and special celebrations, however, all add extra distractions and strange food to the firefight. If there is any time when things will go astray, it is during those events. Working with them is extremely trying but important.

The following paragraphs detail my fun experiences when on the wrong insulin—75/25 Humalog coupled with Starlix or glyburide. These have been provided to give you examples when things go wrong. Normally, one's BG readings should be moving slowly, like the waves on a placid lake. When it changes dramatically in less than an hour or every fifteen minutes, one needs to check carefully the dose and type of insulin and food intake to match up to the Starlix.

Two key issues stand out, namely BG-diet control and stopping the blood sugar from going too low (e.g., below one hundred) and causing the liver to do an emergency glucose add and shoot the BG to 278-plus. As previously documented, the dawn effect is equally broken and results in breakfast BG numbers of 238 to 265 and extra glucose sloshing around my system. In my case, I also get some strange liver dumps that occur when there is turbulence of the BG value where it is decaying and then suddenly reverses direction. The value of the BG is well above 100 and in fact it can be from 140 to over 200 and this happens.

Seeing one's BG get immediately thrashed due to liver dumps and at fun times can really cause stress and heartache. Keeping them tamed is a job for the gods.

Suffice it to say that all this monitoring at special events, vacations, dinners may require Herculean efforts to survive and enjoy.

A low-glycemic story: One bright Sunday morning after a good brunch with friends at a local café, we decided to drive out to Costco and do some shopping. My BG numbers before and after the café were great. I had an omelet, some bacon, and two chocolate-covered fresh strawberries. I had a piece of the fancy coffee cake that restaurants hand out with meals. In any event, there we were at Costco; we walked at least half a mile across the parking lot, and then wandered all around inside the huge store. I had been neglecting my BG and got a gnawing feeling about it, so I took it. It was 92 and dropping. I consumed four large glucose tablets and got it back to 100. After getting through the checkout, which took about fifteen minutes, I checked again and the BG was back at 92. Great. I took two more glucose tablets and after fifteen to thirty minutes, it was back at 104. I stumbled across the parking lot to my car, and the BG was back to 94. I took three more tablets and drove home, checking every fifteen minutes, and it finally got to 140 and higher. In conclusion, I learned that if I intend to do any strenuous activities, I have to be sure to include carbohydrates at meals as that is what the body relies on. If I don't, I will be stuffing glucose tablets.

Another equally unfunny story: "I know I ate properly but what happened to my blood glucose?" Parasites (i.e., giardia) in your gut will interrupt fat digestion, cause diarrhea, and rob your body of the sugars it needs. You need to get these freeloaders out as soon as possible. Watch where you get your drinking water from and properly filter it, if necessary. Otherwise, you will be munching glucose tablets.

Between diet and medications, your blood glucose always tends to throw you a curve. Some days it is too low; some days it is too high; sometimes the digestion cycle is delayed or takes longer (e.g., to process fat and beef). Just because you used so many units of Humalog and Lantus at one time doesn't mean that at other times those amounts could be insufficient or too strong. If my blood glucose is too high, I take quarter-mile walks to bring it down. I had a nightmare after I returned home from visiting my son. I tried to continue my Humalog and Lantus drill, and every day I had two to three crashes due to my sugar going too low and my liver did an emergency add of glucose shooting my BG to 278. I carefully adjusted the Humalog down to 23 units in the morning, lowered the evening dose of Lantus to 10 units, and added snacks for the low zones. After that, I was back on track. Be aware of changes and watch or adjust your insulin, always following your doctor's advice.

As previously indicated, if your liver and its signaling is working correctly, the liver can do any of the above-mentioned Glucose add functions and not flood the system with glucose.

Maintaining your blood glucose between 90 and 110 is desirable, if you can do it. I recommend constant glucose monitoring with a remote display panel. On the wrong insulin and oral Starlix/glyburide pills, if my blood glucose gets below 130, my six-foot, two-inch, 300-pound frame burns glucose fast and causes the blood glucose to drop to 70. On top of that, I would have to be a picture frame on wall, not moving and breathing only slightly. In addition, at these low levels I needed to check my BG at least every fifteen minutes to avoid missing a crash or underrun. So far the only time I've seen my blood sugar stay stable, between 90 and 110, is at night when the insulin levels are very low.

I find it helpful to run my blood glucose below 140 (i.e., 130 to 140) when I am at home resting. When I am running about, driving the car, I push it to 150 to 180 to reduce underruns as well as the need for excessive monitoring. There are times when I was traveling—walking through cavernous airports and the idiotically long security lines, etc.—and the only thing I could do was leave my blood glucose at 180 and bring it down later. Today on thr correct all insulin strategy; this approaches are no longer required.

One of the heartaches is that so many things can twist and throw blood glucose off. Never mind one's own mistakes, such as pills taken late, etc. It gets so tempting to apportion blame, to your mate and others. In the end there is only one person with his hands firmly on the shovel—me. It is just that I get tired of blaming myself.

One of the toughest issues to deal with is that in the past, my body's complex, layered, glucose-feedback systems kept everything under control automatically. Now with this type 2 diabetes, it seems as if the glucose-control systems are on manual, and I now have to use diet, exercise, and food and pill scheduling to get some measure of control. I now am faced with running an old-style steam engine on a new, rigid timetable, and all the flexibility that I once had has vaporized.

Another factor driving me nuts are the blood-glucose meters intended for home use. When they work—and there are no other factors, such as dehydration, other alcohol sugars, etc.—the 20-percent maximum error they get is barely acceptable. I do not mind that the complete meter has a 20-percent error, but that each strip can have up to a 20-percent error is crap. The strips should be sorted to under 5-percent error maximum in a batch. The strips are costly, and I have found many serious errors when I eat out and am slightly dry. The only choice is to retest when the numbers are screwy and do not reflect the human body's response time. Once I was out at a Chinese restaurant and thought, *Great, I will test.* I had two new meters—Accu-Chek and One Touch—and both meters showed super-high numbers that would not clear until I was a half-hour away from the restaurant and had drank a half-gallon of water. Only then did the meters start to work again.

Other than meter issues; as previously indicated, most of the grief over BG numbers and rapidly changing have been resolved by getting on the correct all needle insulin approach and dose with a short duration of five hours. As a result, oral Starlix/glyburide pills dropped.

# Chapter 14

## Insulin Loading and BG Numbers

Whether by needle-injecting liquid insulin or ingesting glyburide or Starlix, which force your body to make more insulin, one has to ensure there is food in the gut to generate glucose for the body to consume. If your liver is working correctly, it can add the necessary glucose to cover this need until digestion takes over. Given my faulty liver-insulin signaling problem, this could result in extra-large glucose adds, to 311 or greater. Thus, for me, avoiding liver add functions was super-critical for preventing bad BG levels and wrecking my averages.

With a needle injection, one has direct control while on a glyburide or Starlix pill, one gets what one gets. Only eating sufficient food will prevent the BG from dropping too low.

The important number to focus on is the duration time of the insulin or pill. On glyburide, you get ten and a half hours of fun on a single pill. If it goes wrong, then you have much less fun for the ten and a half hours. The same goes for insulin. A twelve-hour duration is tough, and you get one shot. Adding more insulin is dangerous as the new charge will add to the previous charge. With twelve-hour durations, this can be tricky and dangerous. Five hour duration insulin and Starlix's four-hour duration enables one to modify after a few hours and make the necessary changes or omit the next starlix pill or reduce or add extra insulin.Insulin provides a dual-edged sword in that when you pick the dose for the meal one ate—for the peak, you need to ensure that once the gut is done, the original value you picked does not take the BG to the basement when the gut is empty. Pick a dose of insulin that reduces the BG peak back to 170-180 so that when the gut completes major digestion, the BG will slowly descend back to 140 (and down to 100, if that is your goal) and go relatively flat and stable.

The BG waveform as seen on the CGMS, as well as averages of finger sticks should be slowly moving and changing. Anything else is a direct indication that there is too much insulin or it was too strong, or the duration time is too long. Should this happen to you, get expert medical advice.

In the past when on the oral pill—Starlix—I usually take the pill anywhere from fifteen to thirty minutes before a meal to ensure a sufficient "ramp up" time for the oral pill. Today, as my pancreas mostly works and except for first dose in early am wakeup, I do not inject insulin until the BG peaks at 180 after a meal , thus preventing extra-low BG levels if digestion is delayed. This saves a ton of glucose tablets. Just remember: taking a Starlix or glyburide pill or an insulin shot before eating means that one must commit to eating food and covering the body and ensuring the BG does not bottom out due to digestion misfire or delay. Add glucose tablets or a snack as necessary.

At the start of an extra breakfast insulin injection and the end of a period of active Starlix or glyburide pill insulin generation, one will want to run BG-meter tests to ensure the blood sugar is not too low when the extra insulin starts up. Otherwise, you will have a race to basement of the BG value. I also used to check near the end of the Starlix and glyburide duration (prior regimen) to ensure there is no premature blood-glucose drop (e.g., if I did not eat enough and the extra insulin drops my blood glucose under ninety).

One day, whoops, I had the trots after eating breakfast. I had ingested Starlix; suddenly I was short on glucose with extra insulin on the loose. This is another reason I test and test often. I had to grab two glucose tablets.

I glance at the CGMS display throughout the day and also do finger sticks. I find that eight tests a day—at 5:00 a.m., 12:00 p.m., 5:00 p.m., and midnight—is sufficient. I stick a finger on each hand, average both readings, and enter the average into the CGMS. Because the system and its sensor looking at interstitial tissue and not fingertips directly; sometimes stumble or foul up, I have done as many as twenty tests in a day. Previously, I had been doing twenty-four to thirty-two finger sticks a day, almost every hour and every fifteen minutes during nasty patches when the gut was running out. This chapter originally had a lot of comments and thoughts about the time I was on the least-appropriate insulin pill regimen: 23 units of twelve-hour--duration Humalog 75/25 and two to three Starlix pills that resulted in highly unstable BG levels that were constantly changing. I include it for reference should a reader experience this and wonder, *What in heck is my body doing?* Get help as soon as possible.

*Notes from my prior mixed meds pre-CGMS experience on 75/25 insulin and Starlix:*

I am a large person, currently at 290 pounds and now losing weight. I had gotten to 330 pounds before arresting this nonsense. One of the things you will run into is the endocrinologist-recommended BG numbers. I am not here to throw stones at that recommendation but to offer my perspective.

The only time I see my blood glucose stable, between 90 and 110, is either in the early morning or late at night when there is no insulin pressure in my body. Typically under these conditions, I will see my blood sugar drop very gradually over three hours, from 180 to 110, based on the small amount of insulin my body releases naturally.

Once there is active insulin present from the Humalog, Lantus, Starlix, or glyburide operation in the pancreas, the chance of seeing that number at 100 or 110 is like a snowball in hell. It either heads to 90 or goes back up.

My personal goal is 140 as an average and a nominal operating point when I am not digesting food. When I see numbers of 120 or lower, that usually means the blood glucose is disappearing faster than snow on a warm spring day. In addition, any chance to arrest the fall will require glucose tablets, immediately followed by a snack. Otherwise the BG will fall too fast for the gut and liver to catch up by themselves. My doctor wants me to keep my BG at 100 or better. This means I must monitor my BG all the time. It is interesting to note that according to the American Diabetes Association, and my doctor confirmed, twice as many hospital patients died maintaining sugar levels at 90 to 110 versus 140 to 180. Typically, when I eat a meal, take a Starlix or glyburide pill, and have active digestion, I will see blood glucose levels of 140 to 180. Above 190 indicates that I've eaten too much carbohydrates or food in general and need to correct my diet in the long term and walk a quarter mile more in the short term to drain off the excess glucose.In addition, when out and about actively doing things, like driving etc., I need to keep my blood glucose up around 160 to 180 to save having to check it every fifteen minutes. When doing intense exercise, I ensure I have extra food and glucose available. The body's normal day-to-day operation does not provide sufficient glucose for heavy exercising, which will flatten blood glucose in a heartbeat.

For many folks, controlling type 2 diabetes may simply involve a better diet, routine exercise, and taking some pills. This assumes your body still has some basal insulin, and the dawn effect and the emergency glucose add work reasonably well (i.e., the liver does not throw a gallon pail of glucose at your body during each of these functions). In my case, they are uncontrolled, and I get the full pail treatment.

Anyone who is more involved with monitoring, the way I am, has now become an engineer and fireman on an old-style steam locomotive and is manually controlling the fuel and water. The size and weight of the locomotive is equivalent to the size and weight of the body. Watching the size of the fire and making sure not to pop the boiler due to excessive steam pressure is same activity involved in type 2 diabetes: getting the blood sugar reduced and under control and not overloading the stomach. When you are not doing much, you will need a bunch of small meals and snacks to keep the stomach operational and ready.

When you want to do heavy exercise or work, you'll need to fire the boiler harder (i.e., provide more glucose so you have enough energy). As a fireman, you are in charge of monitoring the boiler/stomach. The key is not to snuff out the boiler; keep a minimum fire much of the time, and then fire it up during heavy exercise or work. If you watch a large steam locomotive start to move, the first thing you will see is massive smoke from the firebox as fireman ramps up the fire, and the engineer applies the throttle to make the beast roll.

A healthy body does this automatically. In a body with type 2 diabetes, these processes work poorly or not at all, and manual intervention is needed to keep things on track. There is a similar parallel with weight and body size. It is much harder to control a large locomotive than a little yard engine. To that end, it is desirable to keep weight and mass down as much as is reasonably possible, no matter what the so-called recommended operating BG numbers are. For example, air travel today—with the long security lines and walking long distances through massive airports—makes controlling type 2 diabetes miserable. Typically, I will keep my BG at 180 during these "survival" tests and then get that down once the traveling is done. From a testing perspective, I have found that when the blood sugar is 140 or higher, the checking can be on an hourly basis. If the BG gets down to 130 or lower, it can shift so fast that checking every fifteen minutes is necessary to identify direction and pressure. If I have taken glucose tablets and I see the BG moving up to 140, I extend testing to a minimum of one hour. Typically, when the BG is 170, once the gut and liver start to output glucose, that goes on for two to four hours at a stable rate, minimizing the need for testing. Here again, a CGMS can automate and simplify this.

# Chapter 15

## A BG-testing Strategy

I use the CGMS most of the time, supplemented by eight tests a day on a finger-stick machine, at 5:00 a.m., 12:00 p.m., 5:00 p.m., and midnight. I use two strips at each time listed, one for each hand and average; thus, four times a day but eight tests.

On my body, I would see significant spreads between each hand and found that averaging made the best sense. I would scan the CGMS throughout the day and watch for any stalled or delayed waveforms or numbers that seemed higher than they should be. If that occurred, I'd test with finger sticks and enter the new BG into the CGMS.

If you need to do only four strips a day, I recommend doing one when you wake up and then one after every meal at the peak of digestion (one and a half to two and a half hours after ingestion) when there is a maximum amount of glucose in the blood from the gut and liver. When you do a small number of these tests, you cannot really get a feel for the pattern and whether a particular reading is reasonable or not. With the CGMS, you'll see the full trend always and, as such, four to eight test strips to spot check the CGMS is fine. Without the CGMS, and if your blood glucose values seem all over the place; you will need to take many more readings in a shorter interval and in order to t see the trends and whether a particular reading is nuts. If you are not checking lows, my take is that six to ten strips a day may be more beneficial. When I was on Humalog 75/25 plus Starlix and did not have a CGMS, I needed to catch the lows and arrest them with glucose tablets. As such, I ended up with cycles that were fifteen minutes apart, half an hour apart, and one to two hours apart if the gut was up and outputting glucose. This resulted in sixteen or more strips. Bad readings and misidentified patterns were a regular occurrence. In my opinion, this is not discussed intelligently anywhere, but the human body uses the blood system as a transport vehicle for raw materials—oxygen, sugars, nutrients, etc. None of this is tightly regulated as the liver and other organs dump components in the system for transport, and the body relies on the heart pumping the stuff around the loop to mix things up. If you do not take many readings, you may not see this activity. If you have ever driven a car with an overresponsive gas gauge, you will see the needle bounce around from low to high as the contents of the tank slosh around. In the body, the addition of sugar and glucose can cause a similar effect. Most of the time, one wants the average reading, as shown by a highly damped meter that always sits at the appropriate level and does not slosh around. Unless you are looking for a low when the blood glucose is dropping fast, and is less than 90, you want the smoothed-out reading that is typical when the gut and liver are not dumping in a big load.Should you sample one of these concentrated glucose loads in the blood before your heart has time to reboot around the system and dilute the blood through osmosis (as thin blood dilutes down loaded concentrated blood), you can get a heart-stopping reading, from 230 to 500. One might argue that the mathematical averaging should reduce these numbers. Based on my extensive experience, they don't; simple mathematical averaging is not same as blood-time integration averaging, as A1C and other results confirm.The other factor that could affect meter strip readings are interference items. Other sugars, vitamin C, and acetaminophen are suspected to boot readings off at least 30 to 200-plus points. Contrary to some hype from quarters that should know better, I routinely run into food products from big, well-known grocery stores with corn sugars, galactose and other sugars that far too routinely shoot my cost-effective meter's readings through the roof. Such products usually last about four to six hours before they are eliminated from my body. I now keep at least one meter using FAD-GDH technology for comparisons, when eating out, to reduce potentially heart-stopping readings. The FAD-GDH strip technologies are not oxygen sensitive nor pick up on other sugar types and read only the human glucose.

The ability to eliminate bad readings from meter-averaging programs is really needed, and some manufacturers provide that. The defective reading is retained in the meter storage for audit and review but should be deleted from the averaging program. There are also bad strips and strips that do not load up fully. They typically show readings 30 to 150 points higher, and those readings should be discarded. When taking a blood sample, follow the manufacturer's cleanliness instructions and a fresh lancet and ensure that the blood flows easily and generates more than you need. Most of the time when I find myself having to press my finger too hard and only get a small amount of blood, I invariably get a reading in the upper 200s.

So, contrary to the hype and PR, strips do not always provide good readings all the time, every time. As such being able to delete the suspicious readings out of the mix is crucial. My last A1C was instructive in that it had determined my daily average as 155 and the A1C as 6.9. My meter average after removing incorrect readings had been 166. So far, when my CGMS is working calmly and properly, its readings track very well with my FAD-GDH strip-meter technology.

Incidentally, you need to figure out which fingers work best on each hand, although I would not use those all the time, but when you bump into screwy high numbers, you can test the other hand. After walking a quarter mile or exercising, I usually find that the readings on either hand or finger are close, within a couple of points. After sitting or working at the computer, I can see up to a twenty- to forty-point difference between hands. If I catch a transport packet of dense glucose on one hand, I usually find that the other hand or finger is much lower; in some cases, there is more than a one hundred-point difference.

In any event, the excellent advice of one meter manufacturer states that if you think the reading suspect, do another strip test. If it is still suspicious, seek expert advice. And, oh yes, as previously Stated, cleaning, cleanliness, and fresh lancets, as prescribed by the meter manufacturer, are also assumed and expected.

Anyway, my pre-CGMS testing and 75/25 morning insulin regimen plus oral pills such as Starlix details are as follows:

1. 5:00 a.m. Wake up; check sugar and ensure there has been no dawn-effect super-dump. If the BG is 100 to 180, the evening metformin worked. If it is 220 to 265, this tends to indicate missed or failed metformin pills at 10:00 p.m. and midnight.
2. Take Humalog and metformin; If BG too high; wait one hour; then walk six to eight turns, a quarter mile per turn to get rid of the glucose dump and the BG back to 100 to 140 by noon. I watch the BG meter every two turns to be sure I do not under run the blood glucose.

Starlix, which is optional, is taken at breakfast later, typically 8:00 a.m. Generally, I did not need a morning Starlix.

Number of test strips: one to two minimum, plus one strip per loop.

3) Always check the BG during exercise, when walking to store, etc.

Number of strips: one.

4) After breakfast is finished (one and a half to two hours after eating breakfast), the BG should be 150 to 180. If it is too low, add glucose tablets.

Number of test strips: one.

5) Post Breakfast. (If used, the Starlix pill lasts four hours). The low-speed portion of the 75/25 Humalog insulin peaks

around 10:00 a.m. and lunchtime; check at those times to ensure that the BG from the gut has not run out early. On a small and low-glycemic breakfast with small quantities of carbohydrates, it is not unusual to see that the Starlix pill (if used) has excess insulin at end of a four-hour stretch. Based upon an 8:00 a.m. Starlix ingestion, one may see a 110 to 130 BG that falls quickly. May need a small snack between 10:00 and 11:00 a.m. to prevent an under run on Humalog or/both Starlix. Breakfast is assumed to be at 8:00 a.m.; if not, adjust timing on Starlix ingestion time.

Number of test strips: one plus two to three for tracking low glucose and the need to add glucose tablets

6) Lunch at 12:00PM. Check blood glucose one to one and a half hours after lunch to be sure the BG is 150 to 180 and not too low. If it is too low, then it is glucose tablet time. I typically find that if the reading is 116 to 130 or lower, my blood sugar is heading to the basement at high speed due to unused insulin generated by Starlix in the pancreas. There is no time to argue; get one to three glucose tablets on board to stop the race to the basement.

Number of test strips: one to two.

7) Near the end of the lunchtime Starlix's four-hour period, I usually see my blood glucose numbers heading to 100 or lower. Usually my lunch is smaller than my other meals, and the Starlix always runs out between three and four hours later. I need a snack around 3:00 to 3:30 p.m. to get to dinner without running out of blood glucose.

Number of test strips: one minimum, plus two to three for checking low sugar and the need for glucose tablets.

8) Dinnertime: Check that the dinnertime Starlix is up to speed one hour after dinner ingestion to ensure the digestion process working and Starlix and the pancreas have something to work on. Typically, my BG is 150 to 180. If I eat a bit too much (exceed my diet), I may get highs of 200 to 210. I usually go for a couple of quarter-mile walks to knock it back to 180 or less. Assuming I did not overeat, there will be enough action from Starlix and the pancreas to consume sugars. After two to four hours, I usually see my blood sugar fall back to 130 or less.

If not, my BG number will be 180 or higher and continue right out past the end of the duration of the Starlix pill (i.e., four hours). I have to work harder with Lantus Insulin shot of basal insulin to get this down.

Number of test strips: one minimum.

9) Once past the end of the Starlix pill, will need to add a Lantus shot of 15 units at 9:30 p.m.

10) Take metformin pill 500 mg at 10:00pm. No test strip.

11) I take my last metformin pill at midnight and charge to bed. I also make sure my BG is above 100, preferably around 120 to 140.

Number of test strips: one.

**Note:** From the above list of testing, one can see the complexity and testing needed on a mixed regimen consisting of a single day—morning, one shot of 75/25 insulin with twelve-hour duration along with oral pills such as Starlix the rest of the day. The trouble I had keeping track of that strategy versus a whole needle low dose insulin strategy of five-hour hour duration Humalog Lispro five throughout out the waking day along with using the CGMS.

*One Day's Blood Glucose Readings, Pre-CGMS; Humalog 75/25 Insulin plus Starlix:*

| Time | Reading | Comments |
|---|---|---|
| | | |
| 11:58 p.m. | 167 | Midnight reading before bed last night. Prefer below 140 to 120–30. |
| 5:09 a.m. | 187 | Wake up. Left hand, third finger from thumb. |
| 5:11 a.m. | 176 | Right hand, third finger from thumb; extra cross-check. |
| | | Unless on an intense walk, fingers and hands vary in readings. |
| 6:36 a.m. | 202 | Check after one hour. Liver and canned cream in coffee push up the BG. No sugar, no snacks, no food were taken at all. |
| 7:05 a.m. | 188 | After walking dog a quarter mile around the condo grounds. |
| 7:37 a.m. | 168 | Humalog fast-acting insulin finally peaks; drive to restaurant. |
| 8:00 a.m. | 180 | BG rises after a low-glycemic breakfast; no Starlix pill. |
| 9:46 a.m. | 168 | Drive to Santa Barbara and after arrival, check BG. |
| 11:23 a.m. | 140 | Slow part of Humalog peaks; no extra snack from 10:00–11:00 a.m. |
| | | Target: with the right-sized breakfast, correct foods, and no extra calories, breakfast will burn out of glucose around 9:40–10:00 a.m. until BG is 140 or less. Eat small snack of protein and carbohydrates. That may last till lunch but may need some glucose tablets around 11:30 a.m. to 12:00 p.m. to prevent an under run. |
| | | |
| 12:20 p.m. | | |
| | 171 | Lunch. Stop at MacDonald's on the road. Take pills plus Starlix; eat lunch of chicken nuggets (seven for me, one for wife, two for dog) plus four fries and water. |
| 1:41 p.m. | 202 | Digestion's peak. |
| 2:13 p.m. | 199 | Go for a quarter-mile walk. |

| Time | BG | Notes |
|---|---|---|
| 3:04 p.m. | 172 | Go for a second quarter-mile walk. |
| | | Target: with the right-sized lunch, correct foods, and no extra calories, lunch will burn out of glucose around 2:30–3:30 p.m. until BG is 140 or less. Eat small snack of protein and carbohydrates. That may last till dinner but may need some glucose tablets around 4:00–5:00 p.m. to prevent an under run. |
| 4:03 p.m. | 151 | End of Starlix. Finish shopping at Ralphs, 3:20 to 4:03 p.m. |
| 4:55 p.m. | 127 | Preparing dinner. |
| 5:26 p.m. | 127 | Cook dinner. |
| 5:45 p.m. | | Eat dinner. |
| 5:50 p.m. | | Take dinnertime Starlix. |
| 6:23 p.m. | 131 | Complete quarter-mile, after-dinner walk with dog; take half a glucose tablet. |
| 6:37 p.m. | 150 | Dinner digestion. |
| 7:00 p.m. | | Take 500 mg metformin plus heart pills. |
| 7:35 p.m. | 161 | Dinner digestion continues. |
| 8:52 p.m. | 151 | Dinner digestion peaks. |
| 9:30 p.m. | | Inject 15 units of Lantus insulin. |
| 9:30 p.m. | 151 | Digestion continues; Starlix is done; and gut is running down. |
| 10:00 p.m. | | Take first 500 mg metformin pill |
| 12:00 a.m. | | Take second 500 mg metformin pill. |
| 12:05am | 138 | Desired BG target is 120 to 130. |
| | | Sleep |
| 5:12 a.m. | 159 | Wake-up and fasting glucose reading. Start whole new day. |
| | | Desired BG target should be 140 and below. Under 180 passable |

The following pages contains copies of my blood glucose detail as logged by the software of the Nova Max meter, my Free Style Light Meter handheld finger-stick data using the pre-CGMS regimen, and finally the readings from Dexcom's software for the CGMS, showing the latest results under the new all insulin and no oral pills such as Starlix/glyburide in the treatment.

## Self Care Page

**snell, james w**
ID # jim1
Blood Glucose Targets: 100 to 200 mg/dL

### Last 2 Weeks: 12/30/2010 - 1/12/2011
Number of tests: 457   Average tests/day: 32.6   Average insulin doses/day: 2.9

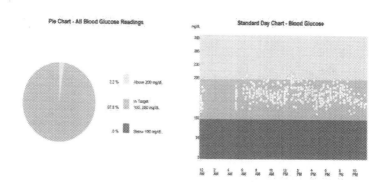

Pie Chart - All Blood Glucose Readings

3.2 % Above 200 mg/dL
97.9 % In Target 100..200 mg/dL
0 % Below 100 mg/dL

Standard Day Chart - Blood Glucose

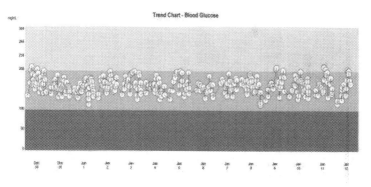

Trend Chart - Blood Glucose

## Blood Glucose & Insulin

**snell, james w**
ID # jim1
Blood Glucose Targets: 100 to 200 mg/dL.

### Last 2 Weeks: 12/30/2010 - 1/12/2011
Number of tests: 457   Average tests/day: 32.6   Average insulin doses/day: 2.9

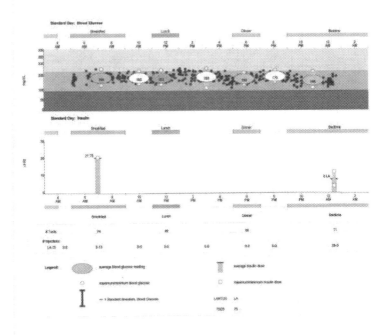

# Self Care Page

snell, james w
ID # jim1
Blood Glucose Targets: 100 to 200 mg/dL

## Last 2 Weeks: 12/30/2010 - 1/12/2011
Number of tests: 457   Average tests/day: 32.6   Average insulin doses/day: 2.9

Pie Chart - All Blood Glucose Readings

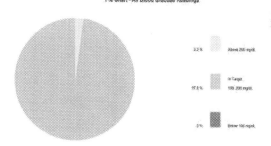

Trend Chart - Blood Glucose

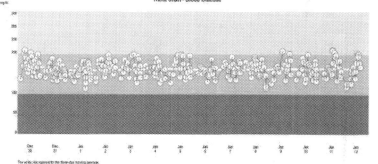

The white dots represent the three-day moving average.

*Jim Snell*

# Summary

**snell, james w**
ID # jim1
Blood Glucose Targets: 100 to 200 mg/dL.

## Last 2 Weeks: 12/30/2010 - 1/12/2011
Number of tests: 457   Average tests/day: 32.6   Average insulin doses/day: 2.9

## Summary - Blood Glucose

| | Total | Avg Tests/ Day | Mean | Std Dev | Min | Max | # Below | # In Target | # Above | % Below | % In Target | % Above |
|---|---|---|---|---|---|---|---|---|---|---|---|---|
| | | | | | | | | | | | Targets | |
| All Unmarked | 457 | 32.6 | 162 | 18 | 114 | 211 | 0 | 447 | 10 | .0 | 97.8 | 2.2 |
| Pre Breakfast | 84 | 6.0 | 164 | 16 | 127 | 209 | 0 | 82 | 2 | .0 | 97.6 | 2.4 |
| Post Breakfast | 42 | 3.0 | 163 | 15 | 134 | 198 | 0 | 42 | 0 | .0 | 100.0 | .0 |
| Pre Lunch | 49 | 3.5 | 163 | 18 | 130 | 203 | 0 | 47 | 2 | .0 | 95.9 | 4.1 |
| Post Lunch | 110 | 7.9 | 168 | 21 | 114 | 211 | 0 | 105 | 5 | .0 | 95.5 | 4.5 |
| Pre Dinner | 56 | 4.0 | 158 | 15 | 128 | 188 | 0 | 56 | 0 | .0 | 100.0 | .0 |
| Post Dinner | 45 | 3.2 | 170 | 15 | 143 | 201 | 0 | 44 | 1 | .0 | 97.8 | 2.2 |
| Bedtime | 71 | 5.1 | 149 | 16 | 115 | 196 | 0 | 71 | 0 | .0 | 100.0 | .0 |
| Night | 0 | .0 | 0 | 0 | 0 | 0 | 0 | 0 | 0 | .0 | .0 | .0 |
| Marked | 0 | .0 | 0 | 0 | 0 | 0 | 0 | 0 | 0 | .0 | .0 | .0 |

# Summary

**snell, james w**
ID # jim1
Blood Glucose Targets: 100 to 200 mg/dL.

## Last 2 Weeks: 12/30/2010 - 1/12/2011
Number of tests: 457   Average tests/day: 32.6   Average insulin doses/day: 2.9

## Summary - Insulin - LANTUS

| | Total Inj | Avg Inj/ Day | Units/Injection | | | | # Days | Days With Doses |
| | | | Mean | Std Dev | Min | Max | | |
|---|---|---|---|---|---|---|---|---|
| All Unmarked | 28 | 2.0 | 8.0 | 2.4 | 4.0 | 12.0 | 14 | 13 |
| Pre Breakfast | 0 | .0 | .0 | .0 | .0 | .0 | 14 | 0 |
| Post Breakfast | 0 | .0 | .0 | .0 | .0 | .0 | 14 | 0 |
| Pre Lunch | 0 | .0 | .0 | .0 | .0 | .0 | 14 | 0 |
| Post Lunch | 0 | .0 | .0 | .0 | .0 | .0 | 14 | 0 |
| Pre Dinner | 0 | .0 | .0 | .0 | .0 | .0 | 14 | 0 |
| Post Dinner | 0 | .0 | .0 | .0 | .0 | .0 | 14 | 0 |
| Bedtime | 28 | 2.0 | 8.0 | 2.4 | 4.0 | 12.0 | 14 | 13 |
| Night | 0 | .0 | .0 | .0 | .0 | .0 | 14 | 0 |
| Marked | 0 | .0 | .0 | .0 | .0 | .0 | 14 | 0 |

Avg Inj/Day = Total Inj / # Days

*Jim Snell*

**Self Care Page**

**snell, james w**
ID # jim1
Blood Glucose Targets: 100 to 200 mg/dL.

**Last 2 Weeks: 12/30/2010 - 1/12/2011**
Number of tests: 457 Average tests/day: 32.6 Average insulin doses/day: 2.9

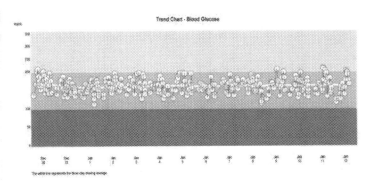

Trend Chart - Blood Glucose

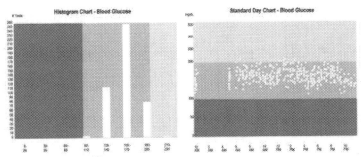

Histogram Chart - Blood Glucose

Standard Day Chart - Blood Glucose

Page 1 of 1 Printed: 1/12/2011

## Summary

**snell, james w**
ID # jim1
Blood Glucose Targets: **100 to 200 mg/dL.**

### Last 2 Weeks: 12/30/2010 - 1/12/2011
Number of tests: 457   Average tests/day: 32.6   Average insulin doses/day: 2.9

### Summary - Insulin - 75/25

| | Total Inj | Avg Inj/ Day | Units/Injection | | | | # Days | Days With Doses |
| | | | Mean | Std Dev | Min | Max | | |
|---|---|---|---|---|---|---|---|---|
| All Unmarked | 13 | .9 | 21.0 | .0 | 21.0 | 21.0 | 14 | 13 |
| Pre Breakfast | 13 | .9 | 21.0 | .0 | 21.0 | 21.0 | 14 | 13 |
| Post Breakfast | 0 | .0 | .0 | .0 | .0 | .0 | 14 | 0 |
| Pre Lunch | 0 | .0 | .0 | .0 | .0 | .0 | 14 | 0 |
| Post Lunch | 0 | .0 | .0 | .0 | .0 | .0 | 14 | 0 |
| Pre Dinner | 0 | .0 | .0 | .0 | .0 | .0 | 14 | 0 |
| Post Dinner | 0 | .0 | .0 | .0 | .0 | .0 | 14 | 0 |
| Bedtime | 0 | .0 | .0 | .0 | .0 | .0 | 14 | 0 |
| Night | 0 | .0 | .0 | .0 | .0 | .0 | 14 | 0 |
| Marked | 0 | .0 | .0 | .0 | .0 | .0 | 14 | 0 |

Avg Inj/Day = Total Inj / # Days

*Jim Snell*

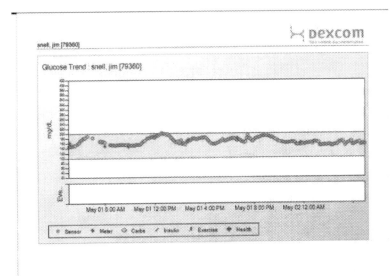

snell, jim [79380]

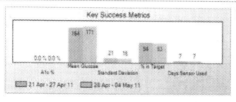

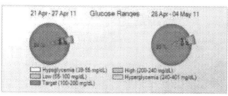

*Jim Snell*

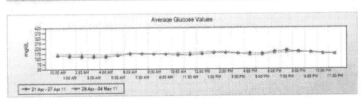

78

⊰ Dexcom

## MySuccess™ Report

| | 21 Apr - 27 Apr 11 | 28 Apr - 04 May 11 | Change | |
|---|---|---|---|---|
| A1c % | 0.0 % | 0.0 % | N/A | |
| Mean Glucose | 164 | 171 | 4 % | ▲ |
| Standard Deviation | 21 | 18 | -14 % | ⊛ |
| % in Hypoglycemia (39-55 mg/dL) | 0 | 0 | N/A | |
| % in Low (56-100 mg/dL) | 0 | 0 | N/A | |
| % in Target (100-200 mg/dL) | 94 | 93 | -1 % | ▲ |
| % in High (200-240 mg/dL) | 6 | 7 | 17 % | ▲ |
| % in Hyperglycemia (240-401 mg/dL) | 0 | 0 | N/A | |
| Days Sensor Used | 7 | 7 | 0 % | ⊛ |

Comment:

# Chapter 16

# Conclusion

I would like to thank the reader for checking out and reading my book. My purpose has been to share my experiences with the monster (i.e., type 2 diabetes), particularly the stroke, recovery, glucose monitoring, and the effort needed to keep the monster in the cage. I may have included too much detail, but readers can select the information they feel applies the most. In addition, there are many issues to ponder and research further.

My biggest goal is to make clear that there is an absolute necessity to actively and properly control and manage the monster, watching all aspects of medicine, food, and diet; exercising; and monitoring blood sugar. It is critical for one to learn about one's own diabetes as well as current cures and thinking in the medical field. Glucose control and limitation through diet and hearty exercise are absolutely necessary for stopping the disease and maintaining good health.

Another aspect that sometimes gets lost is that not all type 2 diabetes patients respond to glucose control and insulin treatment. In my case, the liver was malfunctioning because it was signaling on insulin incorrectly, causing me to have high blood glucose and failing eyes, kidneys, lungs, and other items. Adding extra insulin and super exercise did not stop that. Metformin was super-critical to shutting down the liver's constant need to make glucose all the time, even when it should have been in fasting mode. According to articles and data on the Web from such sources as the Salk Institute and Johns Hopkins detailed earlier, the latest thinking indicates that metformin is way more powerful and helpful in what it does by signaling the liver cells directly and forcing the liver into fasting mode, but that information is not getting out to the public.

In fact, the high glucose levels caused by the liver confounded standard medical treatment, which suggested I should throw more insulin at it. In fact, my impression was that I was overloaded with powerful 75/25 Humalog insulin. Using metformin and lower doses of standard Humalog Lispro, my BG settled down, and I was able to get stable readings easily without having to do thirty-plus finger sticks a day to track it. For me, a good CGMS is critical to fixing tough cases like this and getting to base of the problem and identifying a workable solution.

My ultimate goal is to help you and prevent you from getting a stroke and then going through the long haul of recovery. Type 2 diabetes is extremely sneaky and slow. The excess glucose acts as rot that gets turned loose all over your body—including the retinas, kidneys, liver, flesh, legs, arms, and toes if you do not properly manage it with great care. Your body will do its ultimate trying to prevent damage and keep you limping along, which tends to hide the carnage until it's so bad, the specific organs can degenerate. If you do not understand or cannot easily get BG readings that are consistent and indicate how your body is doing (i.e., the readings are all over the place and make no sense) it is critical that you get help and assistance to solve this problem.

The other immediate action to do is exercise heartily every day, without exception. I walk one to two miles. Diet control is equally important for controlling carbohydrates. Get a dietitian and a diabetes trainer. I did not do that during the early days of my type 2 diabetes, when conditions were slight but ominous. Now thirty years later, after having a stroke, I am making up for lost time. I'm now healing as indicated from results from four different labs, focused on eyes, legs, kidneys, weight loss, pulmonary functions, and heart. My blood sugar numbers are now tracking properly. Another most important issue needs to be stated. Your type 2 diabetes may not necessarily be due to your moral or mental control or be your fault. In addition, your current treatment thus far may be misguided and ineffective. In the later stages after my stroke, my liver was dumping huge amounts of glucose into my blood system. The liver dawn effect shoved the morning sugar up to 235 to 245 and the emergency liver glucose addition during the waking day would increase the blood glucose to 278 to 311. It had nothing to do with the previous night's Roman orgy with a fork and spoon but rather was because of an out-of-control liver and faulty feedback systems in my body.

Type 2 diabetes is a very nasty business; tons of misinformation and well-intentioned but misguided help out there does not help. Determined and persistent effort is required to winnow out the data that can help.